Integrating Evidence-Based Trauma Therapies

A Practice Guide to Multi-Modal Care for Complex Trauma and Personality Patterns

I0039475

Mable Jacquard McGowan

ISBN: 978-1-7642339-5-8

Table of Contents

Chapter 1: The Integration Revolution in Psychotherapy

The field of psychotherapy stands at a crossroads. Gone are the days when we could practice in isolation, wedded to a single theoretical approach while clients present with increasingly complex needs that demand more than any one modality can provide (1). You know this reality. You've sat across from clients whose trauma histories span decades, whose symptoms cross diagnostic boundaries, and whose healing requires something more nuanced than what your training manual suggested.

This integration revolution isn't just a trend—it's a necessity born from clinical reality. When Sarah, a 34-year-old attorney, walked into my office carrying the weight of childhood sexual abuse, a perfectionist schema that drove her to work 80-hour weeks, and somatic symptoms that left her feeling disconnected from her body, I knew that choosing between Schema Therapy, EMDR, or somatic approaches would be like trying to address a house fire with only one tool in the toolkit (2).

The truth is, our clients don't organize their suffering according to our theoretical orientations. They arrive with layered experiences that demand layered responses. This chapter introduces you to a framework for integration that honors both clinical wisdom and empirical evidence—because good intentions without solid foundations help no one.

The Historical Context of Integration

The integration movement didn't emerge in a vacuum. It grew from the recognition that despite the proliferation of therapeutic approaches throughout the 20th century, no single modality could adequately address the full spectrum of human psychological distress (3). The Society for the Exploration of Psychotherapy Integration (SEPI), founded in 1983, became the voice for clinicians who knew intuitively what research was beginning to confirm: combination approaches often yielded superior outcomes for complex presentations (4).

Consider the evolution from Freud's talking cure to today's neuroscience-informed practices. We've moved from viewing therapy as an art form practiced by lone wolves to understanding it as both science and art, requiring collaboration between approaches that complement rather than compete with each other (5).

The data tells a compelling story. Recent meta-analyses indicate that between 25-50% of practicing clinicians identify as integrative in their orientation (6). This isn't therapeutic promiscuity—it's clinical sophistication. These practitioners recognize that rigid adherence to single approaches often fails clients who need the trauma processing power of EMDR combined with the mode work of Schema Therapy and the body awareness of somatic approaches.

Understanding Different Integration Models

Not all integration is created equal. You need to distinguish between what works and what simply sounds good in theory. Let's examine the primary integration models that inform our approach.

Common Factors Integration focuses on the elements shared across therapeutic approaches: the therapeutic alliance, instillation of hope, and provision of a healing framework (7). While valuable, this model alone doesn't address the specific technical requirements for complex trauma presentations.

Technical Integration, by contrast, combines specific techniques from different modalities based on client needs and treatment phases (8). This is where our work lives. When Maria, a 45-year-old teacher with attachment trauma, needed bilateral stimulation to process specific memories while simultaneously working with her protective modes, technical integration provided the roadmap for combining EMDR protocols with Schema Therapy interventions.

Theoretical Integration attempts to create new, unified theories that blend concepts from multiple approaches (9). While intellectually appealing, these models often become so abstract that they lose clinical utility.

Case Example: Elena's Story

Elena, a 28-year-old nurse, presented with what initially appeared to be straightforward PTSD following a workplace assault. Traditional EMDR protocols made sense—until we discovered that her trauma response was nested within deeper attachment injuries and a Vulnerability to Harm schema that had roots in childhood medical trauma (10).

Using EMDR alone would have addressed the recent incident but left the underlying schema architecture untouched. Schema Therapy by itself would have provided the conceptual framework but lacked the trauma processing power needed for the workplace incident. Her body held the memories in ways that neither approach fully addressed.

The integration approach proceeded in phases:

1. **Assessment Phase**: Using schema assessments alongside trauma history and somatic awareness evaluation
2. **Stabilization Phase**: Building healthy adult resources while establishing somatic regulation
3. **Processing Phase**: EMDR for specific incidents combined with schema mode work
4. **Integration Phase**: Connecting new insights to daily functioning through body-based practices

Elena's healing accelerated when we could address her trauma at multiple levels simultaneously. The bilateral stimulation helped process the assault memories while mode work addressed her Vulnerable Child, and somatic techniques helped her reconnect with her body's wisdom.

Case Example: Marcus's Journey

Marcus, a 42-year-old contractor, arrived with what he called "anger problems." His wife threatened to leave unless he got help for his explosive outbursts that seemed to come from nowhere. Traditional anger management hadn't touched the core issues (11).

Assessment revealed a complex picture: early childhood abuse had created strong Punitive Parent and Angry Child modes, recent job stress was triggering his Abandonment schema, and his body held chronic tension patterns that preceded his emotional explosions.

The integration process helped Marcus understand his anger as information rather than pathology. EMDR processing of childhood abuse memories reduced their emotional charge, schema mode work helped him recognize internal triggers, and somatic techniques taught him to notice body signals before explosion points.

After eight months of integrated treatment, Marcus reported: "I finally understand why I react the way I do. I can feel the anger building in my chest before it takes over my whole system. That gives me choices I never had before."

Case Example: Dr. Rodriguez's Transformation

Dr. Rodriguez, a 55-year-old physician, sought therapy for what she described as "burnout that won't quit." Despite reducing her patient load and taking vacations, she remained exhausted and disconnected from the work she once loved (12).

Our assessment revealed that her Self-Sacrifice schema, developed through childhood parentification, was driving her to ignore her own needs while caring for others. Her Punitive Parent mode criticized any self-care attempts, and years of chronic stress had dysregulated her nervous system.

The integration approach addressed multiple levels:

- EMDR processing of childhood memories when she first learned to ignore her needs

- Schema mode work to strengthen her Healthy Adult and soften her Punitive Parent
- Somatic practices to restore nervous system regulation and body awareness

Dr. Rodriguez's breakthrough came when she could feel in her body the difference between healthy caregiving and compulsive self-sacrifice. "I can actually feel now when I'm giving from fullness versus emptiness," she shared. "That physical awareness changes everything about how I practice medicine."

The Neuroscience Foundation

Modern neuroscience provides the foundation for understanding why integration works. Trauma affects multiple brain systems—the limbic system that processes emotions, the prefrontal cortex that manages executive function, and the brainstem that controls arousal (13). Single-modality approaches often target only one of these systems.

EMDR's bilateral stimulation affects limbic processing and memory consolidation (14). Schema Therapy's cognitive and emotional techniques engage prefrontal and limbic regions (15). Somatic approaches directly influence brainstem regulation and autonomic nervous system functioning (16). Integration allows us to work across all these systems simultaneously.

The polyvagal theory helps explain why somatic awareness enhances other therapeutic approaches (17). When clients can track their nervous system states, they become more responsive to schema mode work and EMDR processing. This isn't theoretical—it's observable in session when a client's breathing shifts as they access their Healthy Adult mode.

The Evidence Base for Integration

The research supporting integrative approaches continues to grow. The Tapia study demonstrated superior outcomes for Schema Therapy-EMDR integration compared to either approach alone for complex PTSD presentations (18). Pilot studies examining somatic approaches combined with schema work show promise for treatment-resistant cases (19).

But evidence extends beyond formal research. Practice-based evidence from thousands of clinicians implementing these approaches provides compelling support for integration when done skillfully and ethically (20).

Ethical Considerations in Integration

Integration isn't a license for therapeutic free-for-all. You need solid training in each modality before attempting to combine them. This means obtaining proper certification, receiving adequate supervision, and maintaining competence through ongoing education (21).

Informed consent becomes more complex with integration. Clients need to understand what you're proposing, why you believe integration is indicated, and how you'll monitor progress across modalities (22).

Scope of practice considerations require careful attention. Integration doesn't expand your scope beyond your licensure and training. If you're not trained in trauma work, adding EMDR to your practice through a weekend workshop isn't integration—it's potentially harmful practice (23).

Building Your Integration Framework

Successful integration requires a systematic approach. Start by developing competence in each modality individually. You can't integrate what you don't understand deeply. This means formal training, certification processes, and supervised practice in Schema Therapy, EMDR, IFS, and somatic approaches (24).

Next, understand how the modalities complement each other. Schema Therapy provides the organizing framework—the map of a client's internal world. EMDR offers trauma processing power for specific memories and experiences. IFS contributes parts work and the concept of Self-leadership. Somatic approaches add body awareness and nervous system regulation (25).

Develop decision-making criteria for when to use which approach. Generally, stabilization comes first, followed by processing, then integration. But within each phase, you'll make moment-to-moment decisions about which tools serve your client best (26).

The Path Forward

This integration revolution represents more than a new treatment approach—it's a return to treating whole human beings rather than symptom clusters. Your clients deserve therapists who can meet them wherever they are and provide whatever tools will best serve their healing (27).

The following chapters provide detailed guidance for implementing this integration in your practice. You'll learn specific protocols, decision-making frameworks, and troubleshooting strategies for complex presentations. Most importantly, you'll develop the clinical judgment necessary to know when integration serves your clients and when simpler approaches suffice.

The revolution has begun. The question isn't whether integration will become standard practice—it's whether you'll develop the skills to be part of this evolution in healing (28).

Bridge to Understanding

Integration sounds appealing in theory, but clinical implementation requires solid foundations. Before we can effectively combine modalities, we need deep understanding of each approach's strengths and contributions. Our next chapter examines Schema Therapy as the organizing framework for integration—because you can't build a house without understanding the blueprint.

Key Learning Points

- Integration represents clinical necessity, not therapeutic trend-chasing
- Different integration models serve different purposes; technical integration offers the most practical application
- Neuroscience research supports multi-system approaches to complex trauma
- Ethical integration requires proper training, supervision, and scope of practice awareness
- Evidence-based integration improves outcomes for complex presentations beyond single-modality approaches

Chapter 2: Schema Therapy Foundations for Integration

Schema Therapy provides the blueprint for understanding how human beings organize their emotional worlds. Think of it as the GPS system for integration—without this map, you'll find yourself lost in a maze of symptoms and interventions with no clear direction home (29). You can't effectively integrate modalities until you understand the schema landscape you're navigating.

Jeffrey Young's genius lay in creating a framework that bridges the gap between cognitive approaches and deeper emotional work (30). He recognized what many of us intuited: surface-level interventions rarely touch the core organizing patterns that drive human behavior. These early maladaptive schemas—the deep beliefs about self, others, and the world—form the foundation upon which all other therapeutic work builds.

This isn't academic theory divorced from practice. Schemas represent the lived experience of every client who walks through your door. When 38-year-old David sits in your office explaining his pattern of sabotaging relationships just as they become meaningful, he's describing his Defectiveness schema in action. When Lisa works 70-hour weeks while neglecting her health and relationships, she's living from her Self-Sacrifice schema. Understanding these patterns gives you leverage points for change that no amount of surface-level intervention can provide (31).

The Architecture of Schemas

Schemas develop through the interaction of temperament and early life experiences. They represent attempts to make sense of confusing, painful, or overwhelming situations during times when we lacked the cognitive or emotional resources to process them effectively (32). These patterns become so automatic that clients rarely recognize them as learned responses rather than fundamental truths about reality.

The 18 early maladaptive schemas organize around five core domains that reflect basic human needs gone unmet:

Disconnection and Rejection Domain includes schemas that develop when safety, love, and belonging needs aren't met. The Abandonment schema creates constant fear that close relationships will end unpredictably. Mistrust/Abuse generates expectation that others will hurt, manipulate, or take advantage. Emotional Deprivation assumes that emotional needs won't be met by others. Defectiveness creates shame about being fundamentally flawed. Social Isolation produces feelings of being different and not belonging (33).

Impaired Autonomy and Performance Domain emerges when children aren't encouraged to develop independence and competence. Dependence/Incompetence generates belief in inability to handle daily responsibilities. Vulnerability to Harm creates excessive fear of catastrophe. Enmeshment/Undeveloped Self produces poor boundaries and unclear identity. Failure generates belief in inadequacy compared to others (34).

Impaired Limits Domain develops when children aren't taught appropriate boundaries and self-discipline. Entitlement creates expectations of special treatment and disregard for others' needs. Insufficient Self-Control produces difficulty managing emotions and impulses (35).

Other-Directedness Domain forms when acceptance depends on meeting others' needs at the expense of one's own. Subjugation generates excessive compliance and suppression of needs. Self-Sacrifice drives focus on meeting others' needs while neglecting one's own. Approval-Seeking produces excessive emphasis on gaining recognition rather than expressing authentic preferences (36).

Overvigilance and Inhibition Domain emerges when children learn that mistakes have severe consequences. Negativity/Pessimism creates focus on negative aspects and expectations of problems. Emotional Inhibition produces suppression of emotions to avoid disapproval. Unrelenting Standards generates pressure for perfectionism and harsh self-criticism. Punitiveness creates belief that people should be harshly punished for mistakes (37).

Understanding Schema Modes

While schemas represent deep beliefs, modes represent the emotional and behavioral states that become activated in daily life. Think of modes as the players on your client's internal stage—each with distinct roles, motivations, and ways of responding to life situations (38).

Child Modes represent the emotional states of childhood that remain active in adult life. The Vulnerable Child carries the pain, fear, and sadness from early experiences. This mode holds the raw emotion that often drives schema activation. The Angry Child expresses rage about unmet needs and perceived injustices. The Impulsive/Undisciplined Child acts on immediate impulses without considering consequences. The Happy Child represents the spontaneous, playful, and joyful aspects that may have been suppressed or never developed (39).

Dysfunctional Parent Modes represent internalized voices from early caregivers. The Punitive Parent attacks, criticizes, and punishes the self or others. This mode often sounds like harsh parental voices from childhood. The Demanding Parent pushes for achievement, perfection, and meeting others' needs while ignoring personal limits (40).

Dysfunctional Coping Modes develop as attempts to manage schema activation. The Compliant Surrenderer gives up authentic needs to avoid conflict or abandonment. The Detached Protector withdraws emotionally to avoid pain. The Overcompensator tries to prove schemas wrong through excessive behaviors in the opposite direction (41).

The Healthy Adult Mode represents the integrated, wise, and nurturing aspect of personality that can balance different needs and respond flexibly to life situations. This mode often needs strengthening in therapy (42).

Case Example: Jennifer's Schema World

Jennifer, a 35-year-old marketing executive, presented with relationship difficulties and work stress. Her assessment revealed a complex schema constellation centered around Abandonment, Defectiveness, and Unrelenting Standards schemas (43).

Her childhood included an alcoholic father who alternated between emotional unavailability and harsh criticism, and a mother who struggled with depression and was emotionally inconsistent. Jennifer learned early that love was conditional on performance and that people she depended on would inevitably let her down.

In her current relationship, Jennifer's Abandonment schema activated whenever her partner seemed distant or busy. Her Vulnerable Child mode would feel terrified and desperate, leading to clingy behaviors that pushed her partner away. Her Punitive Parent mode would then attack her for being "needy and pathetic." Her Overcompensator mode would try to prove her worth through perfect performance at work, leading to exhaustion and resentment.

Understanding Jennifer's schema map allowed us to make sense of patterns that had previously seemed random and confusing. Her relationship difficulties weren't character flaws—they were predictable responses from an internal system organized around early survival strategies.

Case Example: Robert's Mode Constellation

Robert, a 41-year-old physician, sought help for what he called "losing himself" in his marriage. His wife complained that he never expressed preferences and seemed to disappear emotionally during conflicts (44).

Assessment revealed strong Subjugation and Emotional Inhibition schemas that developed in a family where his mother was chronically ill and his father worked constantly. Robert learned that his needs didn't matter and that expressing emotions created additional burden for already overwhelmed caregivers.

His primary modes included:

- **Compliant Surrenderer**: Automatically agreeing with others to avoid conflict
- **Detached Protector**: Withdrawing emotionally when situations became challenging
- **Punitive Parent**: Criticizing himself for having needs or emotions
- **Vulnerable Child**: Carrying unexpressed sadness and fear

Robert's Healthy Adult mode was significantly underdeveloped. He had little practice identifying his own preferences, expressing emotions directly, or setting appropriate boundaries.

The integration work helped Robert recognize mode shifts as they happened. "I can actually feel now when I slip into that automatic agreement pattern," he reported after several months. "There's this sensation in my chest, like everything just goes flat. That's my signal that my Compliant Surrenderer has taken over."

Case Example: Maria's Complex Presentation

Maria, a 29-year-old social worker, presented with symptoms that crossed multiple diagnostic categories: depression, anxiety, relationship instability, and periodic dissociative episodes (45). Traditional diagnostic approaches had led to multiple medication trials and symptom-focused interventions with limited success.

Schema assessment revealed a trauma-informed constellation: Abandonment, Mistrust/Abuse, Defectiveness, and Emotional Deprivation schemas stemming from childhood sexual abuse and emotional neglect. Her mode constellation was complex and rapidly shifting:

- **Vulnerable Child**: Carried the terror and pain from abuse experiences
- **Angry Child**: Held rage about betrayal and violation
- **Punitive Parent**: Blamed her for the abuse and current difficulties
- **Detached Protector**: Created emotional numbing during overwhelm
- **Compliant Surrenderer**: Adapted to others' needs while ignoring her own

Maria's dissociative episodes made sense within this framework—they represented her Detached Protector mode activating to manage overwhelming emotion from her Child modes. Her relationship patterns reflected her Abandonment schema creating push-pull dynamics as she simultaneously craved and feared intimacy.

Understanding Maria's internal system allowed us to approach her symptoms as information about her adaptive strategies rather than pathology to be eliminated. This reframe alone created significant relief and hope for change.

Schema Assessment and Measurement

Effective integration requires accurate assessment of schema patterns. The Young Schema Questionnaire (YSQ-3) provides standardized measurement of the 18 early maladaptive schemas (46). The Schema Mode Inventory (SMI) assesses mode activation patterns (47). However, these instruments only provide starting points for deeper exploration.

Clinical interviewing remains essential for understanding how schemas developed and how they currently impact functioning. Ask about childhood experiences, but focus on understanding the emotional themes rather than collecting detailed narratives. Look for patterns across relationships, work situations, and stress responses.

Pay attention to language patterns that reveal schema activation. Clients with Defectiveness schemas often use self-attacking language automatically. Those with Abandonment schemas may express relationship fears in catastrophic terms. Vulnerability to Harm schemas appear through excessive worry about unlikely dangers.

Schema Origins and Development

Schemas develop through four primary mechanisms. **Toxic Frustration of Needs** occurs when core emotional needs are consistently unmet despite being reasonable for the developmental stage. A child who receives intermittent attention may develop an Abandonment schema (48).

Traumatization involves experiences that overwhelm a child's coping capacity. Physical, sexual, or emotional abuse creates schemas like Mistrust/Abuse and Defectiveness. However, trauma isn't limited to obvious abuse—emotional neglect can be equally damaging (49).

Vicarious Learning happens when children observe others' experiences and internalize the lessons. A child who watches a parent struggle with depression may develop Vulnerability to Harm schemas about the unpredictability of emotional stability (50).

Selective Internalization occurs when children identify with problematic aspects of caregivers. A child with a critical parent may develop strong Punitive Parent modes that mirror the internalized critical voice (51).

Understanding schema origins helps predict which therapeutic approaches will be most effective. Schemas rooted in traumatic experiences often require trauma processing through EMDR. Those developed through chronic emotional neglect may respond better to mode work and somatic approaches that help clients reconnect with their emotional world.

Integration Points with Other Modalities

Schema Therapy's strength lies in its ability to serve as an organizing framework for other approaches. EMDR targets become clearer when viewed through a schema lens. Instead of processing random traumatic memories, you can identify schema-maintaining memories that keep patterns activated (52).

IFS work gains focus when you understand the relationship between schema modes and parts. The Vulnerable Child mode often corresponds to IFS exiles, while Dysfunctional Coping modes align with IFS protectors. The Healthy Adult mode parallels the IFS concept of Self-leadership (53).

Somatic approaches make sense within schema theory because schemas aren't just cognitive beliefs—they're embodied patterns that include physical tension, breathing patterns, and nervous system responses. The Unrelenting Standards schema often appears as chronic muscle tension and shallow breathing. The Abandonment schema may manifest as chest tightness and hypervigilance (54).

Building the Healthy Adult Mode

The Healthy Adult mode represents the goal of integration work—a state of psychological functioning that can balance different needs, respond flexibly to situations, and maintain emotional regulation under stress (55). This mode doesn't eliminate other modes but rather provides loving, wise leadership for the internal system.

Healthy Adult functions include:

- **Emotional Regulation**: Managing difficult emotions without being overwhelmed or completely shut down
- **Boundary Setting**: Knowing when to say yes and no based on authentic needs and values
- **Self-Advocacy**: Standing up for legitimate needs and rights while respecting others
- **Perspective Taking**: Understanding situations from multiple viewpoints without losing one's own position
- **Decision Making**: Choosing actions based on values and long-term consequences rather than immediate impulses or fears

- **Self-Compassion**: Treating oneself with kindness during mistakes and difficulties (56)

Building the Healthy Adult requires more than cognitive understanding. Clients need experiential practices that help them access this way of being. Guided imagery, chair work, and somatic techniques all contribute to this development.

Clinical Applications

Schema Therapy provides multiple intervention points for integration work. **Cognitive techniques** help clients recognize schema patterns and develop more balanced thinking. **Experiential techniques** like chair work and imagery allow direct access to modes. **Behavioral interventions** help clients practice new responses outside of session (57).

The therapeutic relationship becomes a laboratory for schema healing. Your consistent warmth and boundaries can provide a corrective experience for clients with Abandonment or Defectiveness schemas. Your ability to maintain appropriate limits helps clients with Enmeshment schemas learn healthy boundaries (58).

Limited reparenting allows you to provide, within professional boundaries, some of the emotional experiences that were missing in clients' early development. This might mean celebrating achievements with clients who had critical parents, or providing calm presence during emotional storms for those who experienced chaotic childhoods (59).

The Foundation for Integration

Schema Therapy's genius lies not in its techniques—though they're valuable—but in its ability to make sense of human psychological experience in ways that inform treatment planning across modalities. When you understand a client's schema constellation, you can predict which EMDR targets will be most therapeutic, which IFS parts need attention, and which somatic interventions will provide the most benefit (60).

This framework prevents therapeutic drift and random technique application. Instead of throwing interventions at symptoms, you can strategically sequence approaches to address core organizing patterns. This is the difference between superficial symptom management and deep, lasting change.

Setting the Foundation

Schema Therapy provides the architectural blueprint for integration work. But blueprints without construction skills remain paper exercises. Our next chapter examines how EMDR's trauma processing power can accelerate schema healing by targeting the memories and experiences that keep maladaptive patterns activated.

Key Learning Points

- Schemas represent core organizing patterns that drive behavior and emotional responses
- The 18 early maladaptive schemas cluster around five domains of unmet needs
- Schema modes represent active emotional and behavioral states rather than static beliefs
- The Healthy Adult mode provides the goal for integration work across all modalities
- Schema assessment requires both standardized measures and clinical exploration of patterns
- Understanding schema origins informs treatment planning and modality selection
- Schema Therapy serves as the organizing framework that gives direction to integration work

Chapter 3: EMDR + Schemas: Trauma Processing Enhancement

When trauma and schemas collide, something beautiful happens—if you know how to orchestrate the meeting. EMDR's bilateral stimulation doesn't just process traumatic memories; it can accelerate schema healing by targeting the specific experiences that created and maintain maladaptive patterns (61). This isn't about adding EMDR to schema work as an afterthought. It's about understanding how memory processing can serve schema transformation.

Picture this: Traditional EMDR targets the "big T" traumas—the car accidents, assaults, and obvious violations that leave clear imprints. But schemas often develop through "small t" traumas—the chronic emotional neglect, subtle criticisms, and accumulated experiences of invalidation that shape our deepest beliefs about self and world (62). Integration allows us to use EMDR's processing power for both types of experiences.

The magic happens when you understand that schemas aren't just cognitive beliefs floating in abstract space. They're embodied patterns anchored by specific memories, images, and sensations (63). When 32-year-old Elena processes the memory of her mother's disgusted face after Elena wet her pants at age four, she's not just healing a childhood incident. She's disrupting the foundation of her Defectiveness schema.

Theoretical Foundations of Integration

Francine Shapiro's Adaptive Information Processing model provides the bridge between trauma processing and schema work (64). According to this model, psychological health depends on the brain's ability to process experiences adaptively, connecting new information with existing memory networks in ways that promote learning and growth.

Schemas represent networks of maladaptively stored information—experiences that were too overwhelming, confusing, or painful to be processed completely when they occurred (65). These unprocessed experiences maintain their emotional charge and continue to influence current perceptions and responses. EMDR's bilateral stimulation facilitates the reprocessing needed to update these networks.

Schema modes often represent dissociated parts of experience related to these unprocessed memories. The Vulnerable Child mode may hold the raw emotion from early losses, while the Punitive Parent mode carries internalized critical voices from childhood (66). EMDR can help integrate these disconnected aspects by processing the memories that created the splits.

The integration approach recognizes that schema healing happens at multiple levels. Cognitive work helps clients understand their patterns. Behavioral experiments provide new experiences. But memory processing addresses the source code—the original experiences that programmed these patterns into the system (67).

The Dwarshuis Eight-Step Integration Protocol

Jeff Dwarshuis developed the first systematic approach to combining EMDR with Schema Therapy for complex PTSD presentations (68). His eight-step protocol provides a roadmap for integration:

1. **Schema Assessment and Education**: Begin with comprehensive schema evaluation using the YSQ-3 and clinical interview. Help clients understand their schema patterns and how they developed.
2. **Mode Identification**: Map the client's mode constellation and identify which modes are most problematic in daily functioning.
3. **Memory Network Mapping**: Identify schema-maintaining memories across the lifespan. Look for patterns of experiences that reinforce specific schemas.
4. **Target Sequencing**: Prioritize memories for processing based on their relationship to core schemas and current functioning.

5. **EMDR Processing with Schema Focus**: Use standard EMDR protocol while maintaining awareness of schema themes and mode shifts during processing.
6. **Mode Integration Work**: After memory processing, use bilateral stimulation to enhance mode dialogues and integration.
7. **Resource Installation**: Use EMDR's Resource Development and Installation (RDI) protocol to strengthen Healthy Adult resources and positive experiences.
8. **Future Template Development**: Create and install positive templates for managing schema triggers in future situations.

This protocol provides structure while maintaining flexibility for individual client needs. The key insight is that EMDR and Schema Therapy enhance each other when integrated thoughtfully rather than applied sequentially.

Case Example: Michael's Abandonment Schema Processing

Michael, a 39-year-old engineer, presented with severe relationship anxiety rooted in an Abandonment schema. His father left when Michael was six, and his mother struggled with depression, becoming emotionally unavailable for months at a time (69).

Traditional schema work had helped Michael understand his patterns intellectually, but he continued to experience panic attacks whenever his girlfriend seemed distant. The schema work provided the map; EMDR offered the processing power to heal the underlying memories.

Assessment Phase: Schema evaluation revealed high scores on Abandonment, Emotional Deprivation, and Vulnerability to Harm. Mode assessment identified a terror-filled Vulnerable Child, a hypervigilant Detached Protector, and an underdeveloped Healthy Adult.

Memory Network Mapping: We identified key schema-maintaining memories:

- Age 6: Father packing his suitcase while Michael begged him not to leave
- Age 8: Mother staying in bed for two weeks during a depressive episode
- Age 12: Mother threatening to "send him away" during an argument
- Age 16: First girlfriend breaking up with him unexpectedly

Target Sequencing: We began with the father leaving scene, as it appeared to be the template for later abandonment experiences.

EMDR Processing: During bilateral stimulation, Michael initially experienced overwhelming terror—his Vulnerable Child mode fully activated. As processing continued, his adult perspective began to emerge. "He left because of his own problems, not because of me," Michael realized. "I was just a little kid."

The processing revealed somatic components—chest tightness and shallow breathing that accompanied abandonment fears. As the memory resolved, Michael's breathing deepened and his chest relaxed. His Healthy Adult mode began to strengthen as he experienced compassion for his younger self.

Mode Integration: We used bilateral stimulation while Michael dialogued between his Healthy Adult and Vulnerable Child. "I understand why you're scared," his Healthy Adult told the frightened child. "But I'm here now, and I won't leave you."

After processing the core memory, Michael's panic attacks decreased significantly. More importantly, he could feel the difference between past-based fears and current relationship challenges. "I can tell now when my old stuff is getting triggered versus when there's actually something to address with my girlfriend," he reported.

Case Example: Sarah's Defectiveness Schema Transformation

Sarah, a 27-year-old teacher, lived with a crushing sense of being fundamentally flawed. Her Defectiveness schema manifested through perfectionism, social anxiety, and a critical inner voice that commented constantly on her inadequacies (70).

Her childhood included a mother with narcissistic traits who alternated between enmeshment and rejection. Sarah learned that her worth depended on perfect performance and meeting her mother's emotional needs.

Memory Network Assessment: Key schema-maintaining memories included:

- Age 5: Mother calling her "disgusting" after a toileting accident
- Age 9: Mother's look of disappointment when Sarah received a B+ instead of an A
- Age 14: Mother saying "I don't know why I had children" during an argument
- Age 17: Mother comparing Sarah unfavorably to her "more attractive" cousin

EMDR Processing Focus: We began with the "disgusting" memory, as it seemed to carry the most shame and self-attack. During processing, Sarah initially re-experienced the humiliation and self-hatred. Her Punitive Parent mode activated strongly: "You are disgusting. You can't do anything right."

As bilateral stimulation continued, Sarah began to access her Healthy Adult perspective. "I was five years old," she said with growing strength. "Five-year-olds have accidents. That's normal." The shame began to lift as she connected with self-compassion.

Mode-Specific Processing: We then used EMDR to target the Punitive Parent mode directly. Sarah visualized her critical inner voice as her mother's face and used bilateral stimulation while dialoguing with this internalized voice. "You don't get to talk to me that way anymore," her Healthy Adult declared. The internal criticism lost much of its power through this direct processing.

Resource Installation: We installed resources of self-compassion and acceptance. Sarah visualized herself as a wise, loving adult caring for her five-year-old self. Bilateral stimulation strengthened this positive resource until it felt stable and accessible.

Three months later, Sarah reported: "The self-attacking thoughts still come sometimes, but they don't stick. I can feel the difference between what's real and what's my old programming. I actually like myself most of the time now."

Case Example: David's Complex Trauma Integration

David, a 44-year-old veteran, presented with combat PTSD complicated by childhood abuse. His schema constellation included Mistrust/Abuse, Vulnerability to Harm, and Emotional Inhibition, creating a perfect storm of hypervigilance and emotional shutdown (71).

Traditional EMDR for combat trauma had provided some relief, but David remained emotionally disconnected from his wife and children. The childhood abuse history had created schema patterns that interfered with intimate relationships even after combat trauma processing.

Integration Approach: We used a layered processing strategy that addressed both trauma types within the schema framework.

Combat Trauma Processing: Standard EMDR protocol for combat memories, but with attention to how these experiences reinforced existing schemas. David's Vulnerability to Harm schema, rooted in childhood abuse, made him hypervigilant to threat in combat situations.

Childhood Schema Processing: After stabilizing combat memories, we targeted childhood abuse experiences that created the original schema patterns. The bilateral stimulation helped David differentiate between past danger and current safety.

Mode Integration Work: David's Detached Protector mode had served him well in combat but was interfering with family relationships. We used EMDR to help his Healthy Adult communicate with this protective part. "I understand you're trying to keep me safe," David acknowledged, "but my family isn't the enemy."

Somatic Integration: Combat and childhood trauma had created chronic muscle tension and breathing restrictions. We combined bilateral stimulation with body awareness to help David reconnect with physical sensations safely.

The integration approach helped David understand his emotional shutdown as a protective strategy rather than a character flaw. As his schema patterns shifted, his capacity for intimacy gradually returned. "I can actually feel love for my family now," David shared. "Before, I knew I loved them intellectually, but I couldn't feel it. Now the feelings are back."

Target Sequencing and Selection

Effective integration requires strategic selection of EMDR targets based on their relationship to core schemas. Not all traumatic memories need processing—focus on those that maintain current maladaptive patterns (72).

Schema-Maintaining Memories are experiences that created or reinforced specific early maladaptive schemas. These often include:

- First memories of schema themes (earliest abandonment, criticism, or abuse experiences)
- Worst examples of schema confirmation (most painful rejections or failures)

- Recent triggers that activate schema patterns (current losses or criticisms that resonate with old wounds)

Mode-Activating Incidents are experiences that created or strengthened problematic modes. Look for:

- Memories where Punitive Parent voices were internalized
- Experiences that created Detached Protector responses
- Incidents that overwhelmed the Vulnerable Child

Resource-Building Memories are positive experiences that can strengthen the Healthy Adult mode. These might include:

- Times when the client felt truly seen and valued
- Experiences of personal strength or competence
- Moments of connection with wisdom or spirituality

Bilateral Stimulation During Mode Work

EMDR's bilateral stimulation enhances traditional schema mode techniques by helping access and integrate different parts of the personality system (73). This isn't standard EMDR protocol—it's an adaptation that uses bilateral stimulation to facilitate internal communication and integration.

Mode Dialogue Enhancement: Use bilateral stimulation while clients dialogue between different modes. The stimulation helps access authentic emotions and responses from each mode while maintaining overall stability.

Mode Switching Facilitation: Bilateral stimulation can help clients transition between modes more smoothly. When a client is stuck in Punitive Parent mode, bilateral stimulation while accessing self-compassion can facilitate a shift to Healthy Adult.

Integration Strengthening: After mode work, bilateral stimulation while clients imagine their modes working together cooperatively can strengthen internal integration and cooperation.

Resource Development and Installation

EMDR's RDI protocol provides powerful tools for strengthening schema healing resources (74). Traditional RDI focuses on developing calm, confidence, and other general resources. Schema-focused RDI targets specific resources needed for healing particular schemas.

Abandonment Schema Resources: Install experiences of secure attachment, unconditional love, and reliability. Help clients access memories or create images of being valued for who they are rather than what they do.

Defectiveness Schema Resources: Install experiences of acceptance, belonging, and inherent worth. Focus on memories or images where the client felt fundamentally okay exactly as they were.

Emotional Deprivation Resources: Install experiences of having emotional needs met, being understood, and receiving empathy. Help clients access the feeling of being emotionally nourished.

Self-Sacrifice Resources: Install experiences of having their own needs matter, being cared for, and receiving without giving. Focus on feelings of deserving care and attention.

The key is matching resources to specific schema needs rather than using generic positive experiences. The bilateral stimulation helps these resources become embodied and accessible during schema activation.

Managing Integration Challenges

Integration work can be intense and requires careful pacing. Some clients become overwhelmed when accessing schema-maintaining memories through EMDR. Others may resist the vulnerability required for deep processing (75).

Titration Strategies: Break large traumatic experiences into smaller components. Process one aspect of a memory (like visual images) before moving to emotions or body sensations.

Mode Management: When dysfunctional modes become activated during processing, pause EMDR to do mode work. Help the client's Healthy Adult communicate with activated parts before continuing.

Somatic Awareness: Pay attention to body responses during processing. Rapid breathing, muscle tension, or dissociation may indicate the need to slow down or strengthen resources.

Integration Pacing: Allow time between sessions for integration. Schema patterns took years to develop—they don't need to be processed all at once.

Future Template Development

After processing schema-maintaining memories, help clients develop positive templates for handling future schema triggers (76). This prevents relapse and builds confidence for maintaining changes outside of therapy.

Trigger Situation Templates: Help clients imagine encountering typical schema triggers (criticism, rejection, conflict) while maintaining access to their Healthy Adult responses.

Relationship Templates: For clients with interpersonal schemas, develop templates for healthy relationship interactions—setting boundaries, expressing needs, handling conflict constructively.

Self-Care Templates: Install templates for recognizing and responding to their own emotional needs, especially for clients with Self-Sacrifice or Emotional Inhibition schemas.

Use bilateral stimulation while clients imagine these future scenarios going well. The stimulation helps the positive templates become embodied and automatic rather than just cognitive strategies.

Moving Toward Wholeness

EMDR-Schema integration represents more than technique combination—it's a approach to healing that honors both the power of memory processing and the wisdom of understanding human psychological architecture. When Sarah can process the shame-inducing memories that created her Defectiveness schema while simultaneously building her Healthy Adult resources, healing accelerates beyond what either approach could accomplish alone (77).

The bilateral stimulation doesn't just process trauma—it facilitates the integration of previously disconnected aspects of self. Clients discover that they can feel deeply without being overwhelmed, access strength without sacrificing vulnerability, and remember the past without being controlled by it.

Expanding the Framework

EMDR-Schema integration provides powerful tools for memory processing and mode integration, but human beings are more than collections of memories and internal voices. We also exist as parts of larger systems—families, communities, and internal family systems. Our next chapter explores how Internal Family Systems work can deepen and expand schema healing by honoring the wisdom and protective functions of all parts of the personality.

Key Learning Points

- EMDR's trauma processing power can accelerate schema healing by targeting schema-maintaining memories
- The eight-step integration protocol provides systematic structure for combining approaches
- Target selection should focus on memories that maintain current schema patterns rather than all traumatic experiences
- Bilateral stimulation can enhance mode work and internal integration beyond traditional EMDR protocols
- Resource Development and Installation should match specific schema needs rather than generic positive experiences

- Integration challenges require careful pacing, titration, and attention to mode activation during processing
- Future template development prevents relapse and builds confidence for maintaining schema changes

Chapter 4: IFS Parts and Schema Modes: Unified Framework

The human psyche isn't a single, unified entity—it's a family system with different parts carrying distinct roles, emotions, and protective strategies (78). Richard Schwartz's Internal Family Systems model and Jeffrey Young's schema modes describe remarkably similar phenomena from different vantage points. When you understand the natural correspondences between these approaches, you can create healing experiences that honor the wisdom of all parts while building internal leadership and cooperation.

The revelation comes when you realize that your client's "resistance" to schema work often represents protective parts doing their jobs— keeping vulnerable aspects safe from further harm (79). That harsh self-criticism isn't pathology to eliminate; it's a Punitive Parent mode (in schema language) or a firefighter part (in IFS terms) trying to prevent future rejection through perfectionism. The key lies in understanding the protective intention behind problematic behaviors.

This integration isn't about choosing between frameworks—it's about using the strengths of each to create more effective healing. Schema Therapy provides clear maps of early maladaptive patterns, while IFS offers respectful ways to work with the parts that maintain these patterns (80). The combination creates possibilities for deep change that honors both the pain of early wounding and the wisdom of adaptive responses.

Understanding the Parts-Modes Correspondence

The theoretical alignment between IFS parts and schema modes runs deeper than surface similarities. Both models recognize that psychological symptoms often represent parts of the personality system trying to manage pain, meet needs, or prevent further harm (81).

Exiles and Child Modes carry similar functions and energies. IFS exiles hold the pain, fear, and unmet needs from early experiences—exactly what schema Child modes contain. The Vulnerable Child mode in schema work corresponds directly to IFS exiles who carry abandonment fears, shame, and sadness. The Angry Child mode aligns with exiles who hold rage about injustice and unmet needs (82).

Protectors and Coping Modes serve parallel functions in managing vulnerability and maintaining safety. IFS manager parts work to prevent problems before they occur, just like schema Overcompensator and Compliant Surrenderer modes. IFS firefighter parts respond to crisis situations, similar to how schema Detached Protector and Self-Soother modes activate during overwhelm (83).

Self and Healthy Adult represent the integrated, wise, and compassionate aspects of personality that can provide leadership for the internal system. Both concepts describe a state of being that can hold different perspectives, make balanced decisions, and respond to life situations with flexibility and wisdom (84).

The key insight is that both models view problematic behaviors as parts or modes trying to help, even when their strategies create difficulties. This perspective shifts therapeutic work from trying to eliminate symptoms to understanding and ultimately reorganizing the internal system.

Case Example: Rachel's Internal System

Rachel, a 31-year-old social worker, presented with what she described as "living multiple lives." At work, she was competent and caring. In relationships, she became clingy and anxious. With her family, she felt like a rebellious teenager (85).

Schema Assessment revealed high scores on Abandonment, Self-Sacrifice, and Subjugation schemas. Her mode assessment identified:

- **Vulnerable Child**: Terrified of being left alone

- **Compliant Surrenderer**: Automatically agreeing to others' demands
- **Punitive Parent**: Criticizing her for having needs
- **Detached Protector**: Withdrawing when overwhelmed

IFS Assessment revealed a corresponding parts constellation:

- **Young Exile** (age 5): Carried terror from parents' violent divorce
- **Manager Parts**: Worked constantly to be helpful and needed
- **Firefighter Parts**: Became desperate and clingy when triggered
- **Critical Part**: Attacked her for being "too much" for others

The integration approach helped Rachel understand these parts/modes as members of her internal family, each with important roles and protective intentions. Her Manager parts (Compliant Surrenderer mode) tried to prevent abandonment by being indispensable. Her Firefighter parts activated when the young exile's abandonment fears were triggered. Her Critical part (Punitive Parent mode) tried to control her neediness to avoid rejection.

IFS-Informed Schema Work: Instead of trying to change her modes directly, we first developed relationships with each part. Rachel learned to appreciate her Manager parts' dedication while helping them understand that constant compliance actually prevented genuine intimacy. She could thank her Critical part for trying to protect her while helping it find less harsh ways to provide guidance.

Schema-Informed IFS Work: Understanding her Abandonment schema helped predict which situations would activate her exile parts. The schema map provided structure for understanding why certain triggers created such intense responses.

After six months of integrated work, Rachel reported: "I can feel when different parts of me get activated, and I can talk to them instead of being taken over by them. My manager parts still want to help everyone, but now my Self can decide when that's appropriate and when I need to take care of my own needs first."

Case Example: James's Protective System

James, a 45-year-old attorney, sought therapy for what he called "emotional numbness." He functioned well professionally but felt disconnected from his wife and children. His marriage was failing because his wife felt like she was "living with a robot" (86).

Schema Assessment revealed strong Emotional Inhibition and Mistrust/Abuse schemas rooted in childhood with an alcoholic father who became violent when James showed vulnerability. His mode constellation included:

- **Vulnerable Child**: Carried fear and sadness from childhood
- **Detached Protector**: Created emotional distance for safety
- **Punitive Parent**: Criticized any emotional expression
- **Healthy Adult**: Significantly underdeveloped

IFS Assessment identified:

- **Young Exile** (age 7): Held terror and grief from father's violence
- **Manager Part**: Worked to appear strong and in control
- **Firefighter Part**: Shut down emotions when overwhelmed
- **Critical Part**: Attacked him for any sign of weakness

The integration approach helped James understand his emotional shutdown as a brilliant protective strategy rather than a character defect. His Manager and Firefighter parts had worked together to keep his exile safe by preventing any vulnerability that might trigger violence.

Building Internal Relationships: We spent months helping James develop relationships with his protective parts. He learned to appreciate their dedication while helping them understand that his current family was safe. His wife wasn't his father—emotional expression wouldn't lead to violence.

Accessing Self-Leadership: As James's protector parts began to trust his Self-leadership, they gradually allowed access to his exile. The first time James felt his exile's sadness, tears came for the first time in decades. "I didn't know I could feel this much and still be okay," he said.

Schema Healing Through Parts Work: The parts work facilitated schema healing by addressing the protective functions that maintained his patterns. Instead of trying to eliminate his Detached Protector mode, we helped it evolve into a resource for appropriate boundaries rather than emotional shutdown.

James's marriage began to heal as his wife experienced him as emotionally present for the first time. "I can actually feel when he's here with me versus when he's disconnected," she reported. "And now he comes back instead of staying gone."

Case Example: Linda's Self-Sacrifice Patterns

Linda, a 42-year-old nurse and mother of three, came to therapy exhausted and resentful. She couldn't say no to anyone—patients, colleagues, family members, or community volunteers. Her Self-Sacrifice schema was so strong that she'd forgotten she had her own needs and preferences (87).

Schema Assessment revealed extreme scores on Self-Sacrifice, Subjugation, and Approval-Seeking schemas. Her childhood included a chronically ill mother and overwhelmed father, teaching Linda that her worth depended on meeting others' needs.

Mode Assessment identified:

- **Vulnerable Child**: Felt invisible and unimportant
- **Compliant Surrenderer**: Automatically said yes to all requests

35

- **Self-Soother**: Used busyness to avoid feelings of emptiness
- **Punitive Parent**: Attacked her for any self-care attempts

IFS Assessment revealed:

- **Young Exile**: Carried sadness about being overlooked
- **Manager Parts**: Worked constantly to be needed and valued
- **Firefighter Parts**: Stayed busy to avoid painful feelings
- **Critical Part**: Prevented selfishness through harsh judgment

The integration approach helped Linda understand her self-sacrifice as a protective strategy rather than virtue. Her Manager parts had learned that being needed was the only way to secure love and belonging. Her exile carried the painful truth that her own needs had never mattered.

Permission-Seeking Protocol: Using IFS principles, we asked Linda's protector parts for permission to get to know her exile. Initially, her Manager parts resisted: "If she starts focusing on her own needs, people will leave her. She'll be selfish and alone."

Educating Protector Parts: We spent time helping Linda's Manager parts understand the difference between healthy self-care and selfish abandonment of others. Her Self could learn to balance her own needs with genuine service to others.

Schema Healing Through Self-Leadership: As Linda's Self gained strength, she could make decisions from Self-leadership rather than protective fear. She learned to check internally before saying yes to requests: "Is this coming from my desire to serve or my fear of rejection?"

After eight months, Linda reported: "I can actually feel the difference now between wanting to help someone and feeling like I have to help or I'm a bad person. My whole family is adjusting to having a mother with opinions and boundaries, but our relationships are becoming more real."

Permission-Seeking for Schema Work

IFS's greatest contribution to schema integration lies in its recognition that change efforts often trigger protective parts who fear that vulnerability will lead to retraumatization (88). Traditional schema work sometimes proceeds too quickly, activating resistance that slows progress.

The permission-seeking protocol asks protector parts for consent before accessing vulnerable material. This might sound like: "I'm noticing that part of you that keeps everyone else happy and never asks for anything. I'd like to understand more about this part and also get to know the part of you that has needs. But first, I want to check— is it okay with your helpful part if we explore this?"

This approach transforms resistance from obstacle to information. When protector parts feel heard and respected, they're more likely to allow access to exile parts that need healing. The protective parts become allies in the healing process rather than opponents to overcome.

Self-Leadership and Healthy Adult Development

Both IFS Self and Schema Therapy's Healthy Adult represent qualities of mature psychological functioning that can provide wise leadership for the personality system (89). The integration approach uses insights from both models to strengthen these capacities.

Self-Leadership Qualities include:

- **Curiosity**: Genuine interest in understanding different parts without judgment
- **Compassion**: Warm regard for all parts of the system, including those that create problems
- **Clarity**: Ability to see situations accurately without distortion from protective fears
- **Connectedness**: Capacity for authentic relationships with self and others

- **Courage**: Willingness to face difficult truths and take appropriate risks
- **Creativity**: Flexibility in finding solutions that meet multiple needs
- **Calmness**: Ability to remain regulated during stress and conflict
- **Confidence**: Trust in one's ability to handle life challenges appropriately (90)

Healthy Adult Functions include:

- **Emotional Regulation**: Managing difficult emotions without being overwhelmed or shut down
- **Boundary Setting**: Knowing when and how to set appropriate limits
- **Self-Advocacy**: Standing up for legitimate needs while respecting others
- **Perspective Taking**: Understanding multiple viewpoints while maintaining personal values
- **Decision Making**: Choosing based on wisdom rather than fear or impulse
- **Self-Compassion**: Treating oneself with kindness during difficulties and mistakes (91)

The integration approach strengthens these capacities through direct experience rather than cognitive understanding alone. Clients practice accessing Self-leadership during session and gradually learn to maintain this state during daily life challenges.

Working with Blending and Mode Flipping

Both IFS and Schema Therapy recognize that parts or modes can "take over" the personality system, creating what IFS calls "blending" and schema therapy describes as "mode flipping" (92). Integration work helps clients recognize these shifts and maintain Self-leadership even when parts become activated.

Recognizing Blending/Mode Activation: Help clients identify the physical sensations, thoughts, and emotions that signal when parts or modes have taken over. The Punitive Parent mode might feel like chest tightness and critical thoughts. The Detached Protector might create numbness and disconnection.

Unblending/Mode Differentiation: Teach clients to step back from activated parts or modes without rejecting them. This might involve breathing techniques, physical movement, or internal dialogue that acknowledges the part without being controlled by it.

Self-Leadership Restoration: Help clients access their Self or Healthy Adult even when parts are activated. This involves connecting with the qualities of curiosity, compassion, and clarity that exist beneath protective reactions.

Cultural Considerations in Parts/Modes Language

The language of "parts" and "modes" can feel foreign or problematic for clients from certain cultural backgrounds. Some cultures view the self as inherently interconnected with family and community systems, making individualistic parts language inappropriate (93).

Adapt the language to fit your client's cultural context. Instead of "parts," you might use "aspects of yourself," "different sides," or "internal voices." Some clients prefer metaphors from their cultural background—roles in a family, players on a team, or instruments in an orchestra.

The key is maintaining the essential concepts—that human beings contain multitudes, that all aspects serve protective functions, and that healing involves internal coordination rather than elimination of problematic patterns.

Building Internal Cooperation

The goal of integration isn't to eliminate protective parts or modes but to help them work together under Self-leadership (94). This requires ongoing internal negotiation and cooperation building.

Internal Family Meetings: Help clients imagine bringing different parts or modes together for discussion. The Healthy Adult or Self can facilitate conversations between protective parts and exiles, helping them understand each other's needs and concerns.

Role Negotiation: Help parts or modes find updated roles that serve protection without creating current problems. The Punitive Parent mode might become an Internal Quality Control Advisor. The Detached Protector might evolve into a Boundary Consultant.

Ongoing Relationship Building: Internal integration is an ongoing process, not a one-time achievement. Clients need tools for maintaining relationships with different parts as life circumstances change and new challenges arise.

The Wisdom of Integration

IFS-Schema integration honors a fundamental truth about human nature—we're complex beings with multiple aspects that all serve important functions (95). Instead of trying to eliminate the parts of ourselves that create problems, we can learn to understand their protective intentions and help them find updated ways to serve our wellbeing.

This approach creates sustainable change because it works with rather than against the natural structure of the human psyche. When protective parts feel heard and valued, they're more willing to step aside and allow access to vulnerable parts that need healing. When exiles feel safe and cared for, they stop driving desperate behaviors that create problems in current life.

Bridging to Embodiment

The integration of IFS and Schema Therapy provides powerful tools for understanding and working with the psychological aspects of healing. But human beings aren't just minds with parts and modes—we're embodied creatures whose schemas and parts live in muscles, breath, and nervous system responses. Our next chapter explores how somatic approaches can deepen and accelerate schema healing by working directly with the body's wisdom.

Key Learning Points

- IFS parts and schema modes describe similar phenomena from complementary perspectives
- Protective parts/modes often maintain schema patterns to prevent retraumatization
- Permission-seeking protocols reduce resistance by honoring protective functions
- Self-leadership and Healthy Adult represent parallel concepts of integrated functioning
- Blending and mode flipping can be managed through recognition and unblending techniques
- Cultural adaptation of language maintains essential concepts while respecting client backgrounds
- Integration goals focus on internal cooperation rather than elimination of problematic patterns
- Sustainable change requires ongoing relationship building between different aspects of the personality system

Chapter 5: Somatic Schema Therapy: Body-Based Healing

Your body knows the truth about your schemas before your mind catches up. That tightness in your chest when criticism approaches? That's your Defectiveness schema preparing for attack. The shallow breathing that accompanies people-pleasing? Your Self-Sacrifice schema in action (96). The hypervigilance that scans for danger in safe environments? That's embodied Vulnerability to Harm creating a constant state of alertness.

Schemas aren't just cognitive beliefs floating in mental space—they're full-body experiences that include posture, breathing patterns, muscle tension, and nervous system responses (97). When 29-year-old Alex describes feeling "small and invisible" during confrontations, he's not speaking metaphorically. His body literally contracts, his voice gets quiet, and his breathing becomes shallow. His Subjugation schema has a physical signature that maintains the psychological pattern.

This chapter explores how somatic approaches can accelerate and deepen schema healing by working directly with the body's wisdom. We're not adding body awareness as an interesting supplement to mental health work—we're recognizing that lasting schema change requires integration of mind, emotion, and soma (98).

The Embodied Nature of Schemas

Schemas develop during early childhood when cognitive and emotional systems are still forming, but the body is already recording experiences through sensation, movement, and nervous system responses (99). A baby doesn't think "I'm being abandoned"—they feel it in their gut, their breathing, their muscle tension. These early somatic patterns become the foundation for later cognitive and emotional schemas.

The nervous system doesn't distinguish between actual threats and schema-based perceptions of threat (100). When someone with an Abandonment schema perceives signs of potential rejection, their autonomic nervous system responds as if actual abandonment is occurring. Heart rate increases, breathing becomes shallow, muscles tense for fight or flight. The body prepares for survival even when the threat exists only in interpretation.

Polyvagal Theory and Schema Activation: Stephen Porges' polyvagal theory provides crucial understanding of how schemas operate at the nervous system level (101). The vagus nerve connects brain and body, continuously assessing safety and threat. Schema triggers activate different branches of the autonomic nervous system:

- **Sympathetic Activation** (fight/flight) appears when schemas like Vulnerability to Harm or Mistrust/Abuse are triggered. The body prepares for action—increased heart rate, muscle tension, rapid breathing.
- **Dorsal Vagal Shutdown** (freeze/collapse) occurs when overwhelm triggers schemas like Defectiveness or Abandonment. The body shuts down—decreased energy, disconnection, numbness.
- **Ventral Vagal Engagement** (social engagement) represents the nervous system state that supports Healthy Adult functioning—calm alertness, connection, and flexibility.

Understanding these nervous system responses helps explain why cognitive schema work sometimes fails to create lasting change. You can understand your Abandonment schema intellectually, but if your nervous system remains hypervigilant for signs of rejection, the pattern will persist (102).

Mode-Specific Somatic Patterns

Each schema mode has characteristic physical expressions that can be observed and worked with directly (103). Learning to recognize these somatic signatures provides early warning systems for mode activation and intervention opportunities.

Vulnerable Child Mode often appears as:

- Contracted posture (shoulders hunched, chest collapsed)
- Shallow, high breathing
- Reduced vocal volume and eye contact
- Tension in jaw and throat (held tears)
- Sensation of smallness or shrinking

Angry Child Mode typically manifests as:

- Expanded chest and shoulders
- Rapid, forceful breathing
- Clenched fists or jaw
- Heat sensations, especially in face and arms
- Impulses toward aggressive movement

Punitive Parent Mode commonly creates:

- Rigid posture with tension in neck and shoulders
- Controlled, constricted breathing
- Tight jaw and narrowed eyes
- Sensation of heaviness or pressure
- Critical internal voice with harsh vocal quality

Detached Protector Mode often produces:

- Numbed or disconnected body sensations
- Restricted breathing and movement
- Reduced facial expression
- Sense of being "cut off" from body
- Cool or absent emotional sensations

Healthy Adult Mode supports:

- Balanced, flexible posture
- Full, natural breathing
- Relaxed but alert muscle tone
- Present-moment body awareness

- Ability to adjust physically to situations

Recognizing these patterns allows for early intervention before modes become fully activated. When Alex notices his chest beginning to contract during a difficult conversation, he can use breathing techniques to maintain Healthy Adult presence rather than slipping into Vulnerable Child collapse (104).

Case Example: Maria's Embodied Healing Journey

Maria, a 33-year-old therapist, presented with chronic fatigue and anxiety that hadn't responded to traditional talk therapy approaches. Her schema assessment revealed strong Self-Sacrifice and Unrelenting Standards patterns rooted in childhood parentification (105).

Somatic Assessment: Maria's body told a clear story of chronic overgiving:

- Chronic tension in shoulders and neck from "carrying the world"
- Shallow breathing restricted to upper chest
- Difficulty feeling her lower body or accessing grounding
- Hypervigilance expressed through constantly scanning environment
- Exhaustion that rest didn't relieve

Schema-Body Connections: We explored how her schemas lived in her body:

- **Self-Sacrifice Schema**: Automatic forward-leaning posture, as if always moving toward others' needs
- **Unrelenting Standards Schema**: Rigid muscle tension and controlled breathing
- **Vulnerability to Harm Schema**: Hypervigilant scanning and startle responses

Somatic Interventions:

- **Breath Work**: Teaching full diaphragmatic breathing to counter chronic shallow breathing
- **Boundary Exercises**: Physical practices of saying "no" while staying grounded and connected
- **Tension Release**: Progressive muscle relaxation focused on chronic holding patterns
- **Grounding Techniques**: Connecting with lower body and earth contact for stability

Integration with Mode Work: We combined somatic awareness with schema mode dialogues. When Maria's Self-Sacrifice mode activated during session (evidenced by forward-leaning posture and interrupted breathing), we paused to help her notice the physical shifts. "Can you feel how your body moves toward me when you start worrying about my needs?" I asked. "What would it feel like to lean back and trust that I can take care of myself?"

After six months of somatic-schema integration, Maria reported: "I can feel now when I'm about to sacrifice my needs for someone else. My body starts that forward-leaning thing, and my breathing gets shallow. That's my signal to pause and check in with myself first. The chronic fatigue is mostly gone because I'm not constantly giving away energy I don't have."

Case Example: Robert's Trauma and Schema Integration

Robert, a 41-year-old carpenter, came to therapy after a work accident triggered severe anxiety and depression. His trauma symptoms were complicated by longstanding Vulnerability to Harm and Emotional Inhibition schemas from childhood with an alcoholic, unpredictable father (106).

Somatic Trauma Patterns: The accident had created classic trauma responses:

- Hypervigilance and exaggerated startle responses
- Chronic muscle tension, especially in back and shoulders
- Disrupted sleep and appetite

- Panic attacks with physical sensations of choking

Schema-Trauma Interactions: His childhood schemas amplified the trauma responses:

- **Vulnerability to Harm**: Made him hypersensitive to any signs of danger
- **Emotional Inhibition**: Prevented natural processing of trauma emotions
- **Mistrust**: Created suspicion about others' intentions to help

Somatic Regulation Building: Before processing trauma memories, we focused on building somatic resources:

- **Nervous System Regulation**: Breathing techniques and grounding exercises
- **Body Awareness**: Learning to track sensations without being overwhelmed
- **Boundary Sensing**: Distinguishing between actual and perceived threats
- **Emotional Expression**: Safe ways to release held trauma emotions

Schema-Informed Trauma Processing: Understanding Robert's schemas helped predict which trauma interventions would be most effective. His Emotional Inhibition schema meant that purely cathartic approaches might trigger more shutdown. His Vulnerability to Harm schema required extra attention to creating safety before processing.

Integration Approach: We combined somatic techniques with EMDR and schema mode work:

- Using bilateral stimulation while tracking body sensations during memory processing
- Helping his Healthy Adult communicate with protective parts through body awareness
- Installing somatic resources for managing schema triggers in daily life

Robert's healing accelerated when we could address trauma at the nervous system level while simultaneously working with the schema patterns that maintained hypervigilance. "I can feel the difference now between being alert because there's actually something to pay attention to versus being anxious because of my old programming," he shared.

Case Example: Linda's Perfectionism and Body Disconnection

Linda, a 35-year-old artist, sought help for creative blocks and relationship difficulties. Her Unrelenting Standards schema drove perfectionism that paralyzed her art-making and created impossible expectations for herself and others (107).

Somatic Manifestations: Linda's perfectionism had specific body signatures:

- Chronic tension in jaw and shoulders
- Held breath during creative work
- Rigid posture that prevented natural movement
- Disconnect from sensual and emotional body experiences
- Chronic headaches from mental strain

Schema-Body Exploration: We explored how her perfectionism lived in her body:

- **Unrelenting Standards**: Created muscular rigidity and controlled breathing
- **Failure Schema**: Produced collapse responses when work didn't meet impossible standards
- **Emotional Inhibition**: Prevented access to the emotional flow that fueled creativity

Somatic Interventions for Creativity:

- **Movement Exploration**: Free-form movement to counter rigidity and control

- **Breath Work**: Using breath to support creative flow rather than control outcomes
- **Sensation Awareness**: Reconnecting with physical pleasure and sensuality
- **Imperfection Practices**: Creating deliberately "imperfect" art while staying present in body

Integration with Schema Work: We combined movement and art-making with schema mode dialogues. Linda's Punitive Parent mode would activate when her art didn't meet standards, creating physical tension and creative shutdown. Learning to recognize these somatic signals allowed early intervention.

"I can feel now when my perfectionist part starts taking over," Linda reported. "My shoulders get tight and my breathing stops. That's my signal to pause and ask my Healthy Adult what would serve my creativity right now. Usually it's taking a breath and remembering that art is about expression, not evaluation."

Breathwork for Schema Regulation

Breathing patterns both reflect and influence schema activation (108). Chronic shallow breathing maintains anxiety states that support schemas like Vulnerability to Harm. Held breath prevents emotional processing needed for schema healing. Rapid breathing can trigger panic responses that confirm Abandonment or Defectiveness fears.

Schema-Specific Breathing Patterns:

- **Abandonment**: Rapid, shallow breathing that reflects anxiety about losing connection
- **Defectiveness**: Held or constricted breathing that tries to make oneself invisible
- **Self-Sacrifice**: Interrupted breathing that puts others' needs before one's own oxygen
- **Vulnerability to Harm**: Hypervigilant breathing that maintains constant alertness

- **Emotional Inhibition**: Controlled breathing that prevents emotional expression

Therapeutic Breathing Interventions:

- **Diaphragmatic Breathing**: Full belly breathing that activates parasympathetic regulation
- **Box Breathing**: Four-count breathing (inhale-hold-exhale-hold) for anxiety management
- **Emotional Release Breathing**: Longer exhales that support emotional processing
- **Grounding Breath**: Breathing that emphasizes connection with earth and stability

Integration with Schema Work: Use breath awareness during schema mode dialogues. When a client's Punitive Parent mode activates (evidenced by controlled, shallow breathing), guide them to breathe more fully while maintaining dialogue with this part. The breathing shifts can facilitate mode transitions and integration.

Movement and Posture Work

Schemas create characteristic posture and movement patterns that reinforce psychological patterns (109). The Subjugation schema produces contracted, small postures that signal submission. The Grandiosity schema creates inflated, dominating postures. Working directly with posture can shift schema activation.

Somatic Interventions for Specific Schemas:

Abandonment Schema Movement Work:

- **Reaching and Receiving**: Practice extending arms to receive support, countering the collapsed withdrawal typical of abandonment fears
- **Grounding Exercises**: Standing with firm contact to earth, feeling stability that doesn't depend on others

- **Boundary Movements**: Physical practices of saying "no" and "yes" with full body engagement

Defectiveness Schema Posture Work:

- **Expansion Practices**: Gradually expanding from contracted postures while maintaining self-compassion
- **Eye Contact Exercises**: Building capacity to be seen without shame or collapse
- **Voice and Presence**: Speaking from full breath and expanded posture rather than hidden, small positions

Self-Sacrifice Schema Movement Interventions:

- **Receiving Practices**: Learning to accept support without immediately giving back
- **Boundary Sensing**: Physical awareness of where self ends and others begin
- **Self-Care Movements**: Actions that honor personal needs and energy levels

Working with Developmental Trauma

Many schema patterns originate in preverbal experiences that are stored in the body rather than accessible through memory or language (110). Somatic approaches can access and heal these early patterns in ways that talk therapy alone cannot reach.

Preverbal Schema Formation:

- **Attachment Schemas**: Develop through early caregiving experiences of safety, attunement, and regulation
- **Self-Concept Schemas**: Form through mirroring and response patterns that communicate worth and lovability
- **World-View Schemas**: Create through consistent experiences of safety or threat, predictability or chaos

Somatic Interventions for Early Patterns:

- **Co-Regulation Practices**: Using therapist's regulated nervous system to support client's regulation
- **Attachment Repair**: Creating corrective experiences of safety, attunement, and care
- **Nervous System Reset**: Helping the body experience safety at a cellular level

Case Example: David's Early Trauma Integration

David, a 48-year-old executive, presented with relationship difficulties and chronic anxiety that had no clear origin in his memory. His schemas suggested early attachment disruption, but he had no conscious memories of trauma before age five (111).

Somatic Assessment: David's body told the story his mind couldn't remember:

- Chronic hypervigilance with scanning for threats
- Difficulty tolerating physical affection or closeness
- Shallow breathing and chronic tension
- Startle responses to unexpected sounds or movements
- Sense of being "unsafe in his own skin"

Developmental Trauma Indicators: The somatic patterns suggested early attachment trauma:

- **Disorganized Attachment**: Simultaneous reaching for and avoiding connection
- **Nervous System Dysregulation**: Inability to maintain calm arousal states
- **Somatic Dissociation**: Disconnection from body sensations and needs

Somatic Healing Approach:

- **Titrated Contact**: Gradually building tolerance for physical comfort and safety

- **Nervous System Regulation**: Teaching self-regulation skills before processing work
- **Embodied Safety**: Creating cellular-level experiences of safety and protection
- **Attachment Repair**: Using therapeutic relationship to provide missing early experiences

Integration with Schema Work: David's Mistrust/Abuse and Vulnerability to Harm schemas made sense within the context of early attachment trauma. The somatic work helped his nervous system experience safety before cognitive work could be effective.

"I'm starting to feel safe in my own body for the first time I can remember," David shared after eight months of somatic-schema integration. "I didn't even know I was holding that much tension until it started to release. My wife says I'm actually present with her now instead of constantly scanning for problems."

Polyvagal-Informed Schema Work

Stephen Porges' polyvagal theory provides a roadmap for understanding how schemas operate at the nervous system level and how healing can support nervous system regulation (112).

Ventral Vagal State (Social Engagement System):

- Supports Healthy Adult mode functioning
- Enables connection, creativity, and learning
- Allows for flexible responses to life situations
- Facilitates schema healing and integration

Sympathetic State (Mobilization System):

- Often activated by schemas like Vulnerability to Harm or Mistrust/Abuse
- Creates fight/flight responses that can feel empowering but exhausting
- May manifest as anger, anxiety, or hyperactivity

- Can be channeled productively for boundary setting and self-advocacy

Dorsal Vagal State (Immobilization System):

- Triggered by overwhelming schema activation
- Creates shutdown, depression, or dissociation
- Often appears with Defectiveness or Abandonment schemas
- Requires gentle nervous system support before other interventions

Clinical Applications:

- **Assessment**: Track nervous system states during schema exploration
- **Intervention**: Support ventral vagal engagement before processing difficult material
- **Integration**: Help clients recognize and respond to nervous system signals

Nervous System Regulation Tools

Building nervous system regulation capacity provides the foundation for all schema healing work (113). Clients need tools for managing schema activation before they can effectively process and integrate new patterns.

Grounding Techniques:

- **5-4-3-2-1 Practice**: Notice 5 things you can see, 4 you can hear, 3 you can touch, 2 you can smell, 1 you can taste
- **Earth Connection**: Feel contact points between body and ground/chair
- **Weight and Gravity**: Sense the body's weight being supported by the earth

Breath-Based Regulation:

- **Extended Exhale**: Make exhales longer than inhales to activate parasympathetic calm
- **Coherent Breathing**: 5-second inhales and 5-second exhales for heart rate variability
- **Bee Breath**: Humming on exhale to stimulate vagus nerve

Movement for Regulation:

- **Gentle Shaking**: Release tension and trauma energy through natural movement
- **Cross-Lateral Movements**: Activities that cross the body's midline for nervous system integration
- **Slow, Mindful Movement**: Yoga, tai chi, or qigong for nervous system calm

Boundary and Safety Practices:

- **Environmental Scanning**: Consciously checking for actual safety versus schema-based threat perception
- **Personal Space Awareness**: Sensing and adjusting physical boundaries as needed
- **Resource Identification**: Knowing internal and external resources available for support

Integration with Traditional Schema Interventions

Somatic approaches enhance rather than replace traditional schema interventions. The body provides information about schema activation, resources for regulation, and pathways for integration that cognitive approaches alone cannot access (114).

Cognitive-Somatic Integration:

- Use body awareness to identify when schemas are activated
- Notice how different thoughts create different physical sensations
- Practice thinking new thoughts while maintaining physical regulation

Emotional-Somatic Integration:

- Feel emotions in the body rather than just understanding them mentally
- Use movement and breath to support emotional processing
- Learn to tolerate emotional sensations without being overwhelmed

Behavioral-Somatic Integration:

- Practice new behaviors with full body awareness
- Notice how schema-driven behaviors feel different from Healthy Adult actions
- Use somatic feedback to guide behavioral choices

Cultural and Individual Considerations

Somatic work must be adapted to individual and cultural differences in body awareness, expression, and healing practices (115). Some cultures have rich traditions of embodied healing, while others may view body focus as inappropriate or uncomfortable.

Cultural Adaptations:

- Respect cultural norms about physical contact, body exposure, and emotional expression
- Incorporate traditional healing practices that include somatic awareness
- Adapt language to fit cultural concepts of mind-body connection

Individual Differences:

- Consider trauma history that may make body focus triggering
- Respect different learning styles and somatic awareness levels
- Modify practices for physical limitations or disabilities

Building Somatic Safety:

- Start with minimal body awareness and gradually increase
- Always maintain client choice and control over somatic interventions
- Provide psychoeducation about the role of body awareness in healing

The Wisdom of Embodied Healing

Somatic approaches to schema healing honor a fundamental truth—human beings are embodied creatures whose psychological patterns are inseparable from physical experience (116). Lasting change requires integration across all levels of human functioning: cognitive, emotional, relational, and somatic.

The body holds both the wounds and the wisdom needed for healing. Schemas may be maintained by nervous system patterns, but the nervous system also has innate capacity for regulation, healing, and growth. When we learn to listen to the body's signals and support its natural healing processes, schema transformation accelerates beyond what purely mental approaches can achieve.

Clients often describe somatic-schema integration as "finally feeling like myself" or "being at home in my own body." These aren't poetic metaphors—they reflect the embodied experience of nervous system regulation and schema healing working together to create wholeness.

Building Practical Integration

Understanding the somatic foundations of schema patterns provides crucial insights for healing, but integration requires practical frameworks for combining these approaches in actual clinical practice. Our next chapter examines specific protocols and structures for implementing integrated schema therapy in real-world therapeutic settings.

Key Learning Points

- Schemas are embodied patterns that include nervous system responses, posture, breathing, and muscle tension
- Each schema mode has characteristic somatic signatures that can be recognized and worked with directly
- Polyvagal theory explains how schemas operate at the nervous system level and provides intervention targets
- Breathing patterns both reflect and influence schema activation, offering direct intervention opportunities
- Movement and posture work can shift schema patterns by changing physical positioning and body awareness
- Developmental trauma often requires somatic approaches to access preverbal patterns stored in the body
- Nervous system regulation provides the foundation for all schema healing work
- Somatic approaches enhance traditional schema interventions rather than replacing them
- Cultural and individual factors must be considered in adapting somatic approaches to schema work

Chapter 6: Practical Integration Protocols

Integration without structure becomes therapeutic chaos. You need clear protocols that guide decision-making, session planning, and treatment sequencing—otherwise you'll find yourself drowning in a sea of excellent techniques with no map for navigation (117). This chapter provides practical frameworks that transform theoretical integration into effective clinical practice.

The art of integration lies in knowing which tool to use when, how to transition between approaches smoothly, and how to maintain therapeutic coherence while drawing from multiple modalities. When Jennifer, a 31-year-old teacher with complex PTSD, needs EMDR processing for traumatic memories while her Self-Sacrifice schema demands attention and her nervous system requires regulation, you need more than good intentions—you need systematic protocols.

Think of these frameworks as clinical GPS systems. They don't make decisions for you, but they provide navigation support when the territory gets complex. The protocols in this chapter have been tested in real clinical practice with hundreds of clients presenting everything from straightforward schema patterns to complex developmental trauma (118).

The Master Integration Framework

Effective integration follows predictable phases that build upon each other. Rushing to processing before establishing safety creates retraumatization. Attempting integration before processing maintains fragmentation. The master framework provides structure while maintaining flexibility for individual client needs (119).

Phase 1: Assessment and Stabilization (Sessions 1-6)

- Comprehensive schema assessment using standardized measures and clinical interview
- Trauma history evaluation with attention to developmental timing and impact
- Nervous system assessment and regulation capacity building
- Safety and stability establishment across all modalities
- Treatment planning with clear integration rationale

Phase 2: Processing and Mode Work (Sessions 7-20)

- Targeted memory processing using EMDR for schema-maintaining experiences
- Schema mode identification and dialogue work
- Parts work using IFS principles for internal system negotiation
- Somatic processing of embodied patterns and nervous system responses
- Integration of insights and experiences across modalities

Phase 3: Integration and Implementation (Sessions 21-30)

- Daily life application of new patterns and skills
- Relationship and career integration of schema changes
- Relapse prevention and maintenance planning
- Future template development for ongoing growth
- Termination planning with booster session scheduling

This framework isn't rigid—some clients need extended stabilization phases, others are ready for processing work earlier. The key is maintaining the sequence of safety, processing, and integration rather than jumping randomly between approaches (120).

Assessment Phase Integration

Comprehensive assessment sets the foundation for effective integration. You need information about schema patterns, trauma history, nervous system functioning, and client readiness for different types of intervention (121).

Schema Assessment Protocol:

- **Young Schema Questionnaire (YSQ-3)**: Standardized measurement of 18 early maladaptive schemas
- **Schema Mode Inventory (SMI)**: Assessment of mode activation patterns
- **Clinical Schema Interview**: Exploration of schema origins and current impact
- **Schema Triggering Diary**: Week-long tracking of schema activation in daily life

Trauma Assessment Framework:

- **ACE Score (Adverse Childhood Experiences)**: Standardized assessment of early trauma
- **Trauma Timeline**: Chronological mapping of significant traumatic experiences
- **EMDR Readiness Assessment**: Evaluation of stability and resources for memory processing
- **Dissociation Screening**: Assessment for dissociative responses that require special considerations

Nervous System Evaluation:

- **Window of Tolerance Assessment**: Evaluation of arousal regulation capacity
- **Polyvagal State Tracking**: Identification of nervous system response patterns
- **Somatic Awareness Scale**: Assessment of body awareness and comfort levels
- **Regulation Resources Inventory**: Current coping strategies and support systems

Integration Readiness Factors:

- Previous therapy experience and outcomes
- Current life stability and support systems
- Motivation and commitment to integration work

- Cognitive and emotional processing capacity
- Cultural factors that influence treatment approach

Case Example: Marcus's Assessment Journey

Marcus, a 44-year-old construction worker, presented with anger outbursts, relationship problems, and work difficulties following a divorce. His intake revealed complexity that required careful assessment (122).

Initial Presentation: "I lose my temper over stupid things, and it's ruining my life. My ex-wife says I need anger management, but I've tried that twice and it doesn't stick."

Schema Assessment Results:

- **High Scores**: Abandonment (85th percentile), Mistrust/Abuse (78th percentile), Defectiveness (82nd percentile)
- **Moderate Scores**: Vulnerability to Harm, Emotional Inhibition, Unrelenting Standards
- **Mode Profile**: Strong Angry Child and Punitive Parent modes, underdeveloped Healthy Adult

Trauma History Discovery:

- Childhood physical abuse by alcoholic father
- Emotional neglect from overwhelmed mother
- Bullying at school with no family support
- Combat exposure during military service
- Recent divorce triggered by explosive anger episodes

Nervous System Assessment:

- Chronic hypervigilance and exaggerated startle responses
- Rapid escalation from calm to rage with little warning
- Difficulty accessing calm states even in safe environments
- Limited body awareness or somatic regulation skills

Integration Planning: Marcus's assessment revealed that anger management had failed because it addressed surface behaviors without touching the underlying schema patterns and trauma responses. The integration approach would need to:

1. Build nervous system regulation skills before processing work
2. Address childhood trauma that created schema patterns
3. Work with Angry Child and Punitive Parent modes
4. Process combat trauma within schema framework
5. Develop Healthy Adult resources for daily life management

"Finally, someone gets that this isn't just an anger problem," Marcus said after the assessment feedback session. "I can see now why the anger management classes didn't work. We were trying to control the explosion without understanding what lights the fuse."

Session Structure Options

Integration sessions require more time and flexibility than traditional therapy formats. Different session structures serve different purposes and client needs (123).

50-Minute Integration Sessions:

- Best for: Maintenance work, specific skill building, check-ins
- Structure: 10 minutes check-in, 30 minutes focused work, 10 minutes integration and planning
- Limitations: Insufficient time for deep processing or complex integration work

90-Minute Integration Sessions (Recommended Standard):

- Best for: Most integration work, memory processing, mode work
- Structure: 15 minutes check-in and grounding, 60 minutes main work, 15 minutes integration and stabilization
- Advantages: Adequate time for activation, processing, and regulation without rushing

3-Hour Intensive Sessions:

- Best for: Complex trauma processing, major breakthroughs, stuck patterns
- Structure: Multiple cycles of activation, processing, and integration with breaks
- Requirements: Skilled clinician, appropriate client selection, careful preparation

Day-Long or Weekend Intensives:

- Best for: Motivated clients with limited time availability, major life transitions
- Structure: Extended processing with overnight integration time
- Considerations: Requires specialized training and careful client preparation

The 90-minute format provides optimal balance between depth and safety for most integration work. Shorter sessions often feel rushed, while longer sessions can overwhelm clients who aren't prepared for intensive work (124).

Case Example: Lisa's Session Structure Evolution

Lisa, a 29-year-old nurse, initially requested traditional 50-minute sessions due to scheduling constraints. Her Self-Sacrifice and Emotional Deprivation schemas created patterns that interfered with the depth needed for integration work (125).

Initial 50-Minute Sessions: Lisa would arrive, briefly mention current stressors, then spend most of the session helping me understand other people's problems rather than focusing on her own patterns. When we approached emotional material, she would quickly shift back to caretaking mode. Sessions felt superficial and frustrating for both of us.

Transition to 90-Minute Format: After explaining the rationale for longer sessions, Lisa agreed to try the extended format. The additional time allowed:

- 15 minutes for Lisa to transition from caretaking mode into therapy space
- 60 minutes for deep exploration without watching the clock
- 15 minutes for integration and planning without rushing

Session Flow Improvement: The longer format allowed Lisa to:

- Notice when her Self-Sacrifice mode activated during session
- Stay with emotional material long enough for processing
- Practice new responses without feeling hurried
- Leave sessions feeling complete rather than interrupted

"The 90-minute sessions feel completely different," Lisa reported. "I can actually get somewhere instead of just touching the surface. I didn't realize how much time it takes me to shift from taking care of everyone else to focusing on myself."

Transition Techniques

Smooth transitions between modalities prevent fragmentation and maintain therapeutic coherence. Abrupt shifts from cognitive work to somatic awareness can feel jarring and disruptive. Skillful transitions maintain connection while shifting focus (126).

Cognitive to Somatic Transitions:

- "Let's pause and notice what's happening in your body as we talk about this..."
- "I'm curious about how this conversation is landing in your physical experience..."
- "Can you feel where that thought lives in your body?"

Somatic to Emotional Transitions:

- "What emotion wants to be expressed through this body sensation?"
- "If this tightness in your chest could speak, what would it say?"
- "Let's give voice to what your body is communicating..."

Emotional to Cognitive Transitions:

- "As you stay with this feeling, what thoughts or beliefs emerge?"
- "What meaning are you making of this emotional experience?"
- "How does this connect to patterns we've been exploring?"

Processing to Integration Transitions:

- "Let's step back and notice what shifted during that processing..."
- "How does this new understanding change your perspective on the situation?"
- "What would you like to remember from this experience?"

Case Example: David's Transition Mastery

David, a 38-year-old therapist, was skilled at intellectual understanding but struggled with emotional and somatic awareness. Learning to transition between modalities became crucial for his integration work (127).

Initial Challenges: David would analyze his patterns brilliantly but remain disconnected from emotional and physical experience. When I attempted direct transitions to body awareness, he would intellectualize the sensations rather than experiencing them.

Bridge-Building Approach: We developed transitional language that honored his cognitive strengths while inviting deeper experience:

- "Your mind has mapped this pattern clearly. Now let's invite your body's wisdom to add information..."

- "You understand this intellectually. What would it be like to know it in your whole being?"
- "Let's use your analytical skills to explore what's happening below the neck..."

Gradual Integration: Over time, David learned to move fluidly between cognitive understanding, emotional awareness, and somatic experience. He described the integration as "finally having access to my whole intelligence instead of just my head."

Documentation and Progress Tracking

Integration work requires documentation systems that capture progress across multiple modalities. Traditional progress notes often miss the complexity of integrated approaches (128).

Multi-Modal Progress Tracking:

- **Schema Changes**: Shifts in schema intensity and activation patterns
- **Trauma Processing**: EMDR targets completed and integration status
- **Mode Development**: Strengthening of Healthy Adult and integration of other modes
- **Nervous System Regulation**: Improvements in regulation capacity and recovery time
- **Daily Life Application**: Implementation of skills and insights in real-world situations

Session Documentation Framework:

- **Opening Assessment**: Current schema activation, nervous system state, daily life challenges
- **Main Work**: Modalities used, specific interventions, client responses and insights
- **Integration**: Connections made between approaches, homework assignments, preparation for next session

- **Risk Assessment**: Safety considerations, crisis planning, referral needs

Outcome Measurement:

- **Pre/Post Schema Assessments**: YSQ-3 and SMI scores at regular intervals
- **Functional Improvement Measures**: Work, relationship, and daily functioning indicators
- **Client Self-Report**: Subjective experience of change and satisfaction with progress
- **Behavioral Observations**: Mode transitions, regulation capacity, integration demonstrations

Homework and Between-Session Integration

Integration happens between sessions as much as during them. Clients need specific practices that support ongoing change and prevent regression to old patterns (129).

Schema Awareness Practices:

- **Daily Schema Check-ins**: Brief self-assessment of schema activation and triggers
- **Mode Journaling**: Tracking mode shifts and practicing Healthy Adult responses
- **Trigger Response Planning**: Predetermined strategies for managing common schema triggers

Somatic Integration Homework:

- **Breathing Practices**: Daily nervous system regulation through breathwork
- **Body Awareness Exercises**: Gradual expansion of somatic awareness and comfort
- **Movement Practices**: Yoga, walking, or other activities that support embodied integration

Relationship Integration Work:

- **Communication Experiments**: Practicing new responses in low-stakes situations
- **Boundary Setting Practice**: Gradual implementation of healthy boundaries
- **Intimacy Building**: Increasing emotional availability and authentic expression

Crisis Management Planning:

- **Early Warning Systems**: Recognition of escalation patterns before crisis points
- **Self-Soothing Toolkits**: Accessible regulation strategies for difficult moments
- **Support System Activation**: Clear plans for when additional help is needed

Managing Complex Case Scenarios

Integration work attracts complex cases that challenge standard protocols. Clients with multiple diagnoses, severe trauma histories, or significant life stressors require adapted approaches (130).

High-Risk Presentations:

- Suicidal ideation or self-harm behaviors
- Active substance abuse or addiction
- Severe dissociation or psychotic features
- Domestic violence or ongoing trauma exposure
- Severe personality disorder presentations

Protocol Adaptations for Complexity:

- **Extended Stabilization**: More time spent building safety and regulation before processing
- **Team Approach**: Coordination with psychiatrists, addiction counselors, case managers

- **Crisis Planning**: Detailed safety plans with multiple intervention levels
- **Titrated Processing**: Smaller doses of integration work with more stabilization time
- **Family System Integration**: Including supportive family members in treatment planning

Case Example: Amanda's Complex Integration

Amanda, a 34-year-old artist, presented with multiple trauma histories, severe dissociation, active eating disorder behaviors, and suicidal ideation. Her schema constellation included almost every early maladaptive schema (131).

Risk Assessment: Amanda required careful evaluation of readiness for integration work given her complex presentation. Standard protocols needed significant adaptation for safety.

Modified Integration Approach:

- **Extended Assessment Phase**: Three months of stabilization before any processing work
- **Team Coordination**: Collaboration with psychiatrist for medication management and nutritionist for eating disorder support
- **Titrated Integration**: Very small doses of emotional processing with extensive stabilization between sessions
- **Crisis Management**: Detailed safety planning with multiple intervention levels
- **Support System Building**: Family education and couple's work to strengthen external resources

Gradual Integration Success: Over 18 months, Amanda gradually built capacity for integration work. Her early schema patterns began shifting as she developed internal safety and external support.

"I never thought I could feel safe enough to look at my trauma," Amanda shared. "The slow approach felt frustrating at first, but now I can see it was necessary. I couldn't have handled deep processing work without building all these safety resources first."

Quality Assurance and Supervision

Integration work requires ongoing supervision and quality assurance to maintain safety and effectiveness. The complexity of multiple modalities increases the risk of errors in judgment or technique (132).

Supervision Requirements:

- **Individual Supervision**: Regular consultation with supervisor trained in integration approaches
- **Group Consultation**: Peer supervision with other integration practitioners
- **Ongoing Training**: Continuing education in each component modality
- **Personal Therapy**: Integration work for the therapist to understand the process experientially

Quality Markers:

- **Client Safety**: Maintained throughout all phases of integration work
- **Coherent Rationale**: Clear logic for modality selection and treatment planning
- **Measurable Progress**: Documented improvement across multiple functioning areas
- **Client Satisfaction**: Positive therapeutic alliance and treatment satisfaction
- **Therapist Competence**: Demonstrated skill in each component modality

Building Your Integration Practice

Developing competence in integration work requires systematic skill building and careful practice development. You can't master integration by attending weekend workshops—it requires dedicated training and supervised practice (133).

Training Pathway Recommendations:

1. **Foundation Skills**: Competence in each individual modality (Schema Therapy, EMDR, IFS, Somatic Approaches)
2. **Integration Training**: Specialized workshops in integration approaches
3. **Supervised Practice**: Mentorship with experienced integration practitioners
4. **Ongoing Education**: Regular continuing education and skill updates
5. **Personal Integration Work**: Experience integration as a client to understand the process

Practice Development Considerations:

- **Client Selection**: Start with less complex cases while building integration skills
- **Session Structure**: Implement 90-minute sessions for adequate integration time
- **Documentation Systems**: Develop tracking methods for multi-modal progress
- **Referral Network**: Build relationships with specialists for complex case consultation
- **Outcome Tracking**: Measure effectiveness to refine and improve approaches

Moving Forward Systematically

Integration protocols provide the roadmap, but effective implementation requires understanding how to create comprehensive case formulations that guide treatment planning across all modalities. Our next chapter examines the art and science of multi-modal case conceptualization—the foundation that makes integration possible.

Key Learning Points

- Effective integration requires structured protocols that guide decision-making and treatment sequencing
- Assessment must be comprehensive across all modalities to inform integration planning
- Session structure significantly impacts integration effectiveness, with 90-minute sessions providing optimal balance
- Smooth transitions between modalities maintain therapeutic coherence and prevent fragmentation
- Documentation systems must capture progress across multiple domains and approaches
- Between-session integration work is crucial for maintaining progress and preventing regression
- Complex cases require protocol adaptations with emphasis on safety and stabilization
- Quality assurance through supervision and ongoing training ensures effective integration practice

Chapter 7: Case Formulation Across Modalities

The moment you sit across from a new client, your mind starts building a story—but not just any story. You're constructing a multi-dimensional map that needs to make sense of their pain while pointing toward healing possibilities (134). Case formulation in integration work isn't about checking boxes or filling out forms. It's about creating a living document that honors the complexity of human experience while providing clear direction for change.

Think about Maria, sitting in your office describing her "impossible" relationship with her teenage daughter. She talks about feeling like a failure as a mother, working 60-hour weeks to prove her worth, and lying awake at night with chest pains that doctors can't explain. Your job isn't to choose between her schemas, her trauma history, or her somatic symptoms—it's to understand how they all connect and inform each other (135).

Traditional case formulation often feels like trying to capture a symphony by describing only the violin section. Integration formulation requires you to hear the whole orchestra—cognitive patterns, emotional themes, body responses, family systems, cultural context, and spiritual connections. This chapter provides frameworks for creating formulations that capture this richness while remaining clinically useful.

The Architecture of Integration Formulation

Effective integration formulation builds in layers, like constructing a house. You need a solid foundation before adding walls, and you need walls before installing the roof. Each layer provides essential information while building toward a coherent whole (136).

Layer 1: Presenting Concerns and Life Context Start with what brought your client to your office, but expand beyond symptoms to understand their life situation. How do their concerns impact relationships, work, health, and daily functioning? What cultural, spiritual, and family factors shape their experience?

Layer 2: Schema Architecture Map their early maladaptive schemas and understand how these patterns developed. Which schemas are most active? How do they interact with each other? What triggers activate them in current life?

Layer 3: Trauma and Memory Networks Identify traumatic experiences across the lifespan and understand how they connect to current difficulties. Look for patterns of experiences rather than isolated incidents. How does their trauma history maintain schema patterns?

Layer 4: Mode and Parts Constellation Understand their internal system—which modes or parts are most active, protective, or wounded? How do different aspects of their personality interact? What does their internal communication look like?

Layer 5: Somatic and Nervous System Patterns Explore how their schemas and trauma live in their body. What are their characteristic nervous system responses? How does their breathing, posture, and muscle tension reflect their psychological patterns?

Layer 6: Strengths and Resources Identify existing capacities, support systems, and positive experiences that can support healing. What's already working in their life? Where do you see evidence of their Healthy Adult or Self-leadership?

Case Example: Robert's Multi-Layered Formulation

Robert, a 42-year-old engineer, sought therapy after his wife threatened divorce unless he addressed his "emotional unavailability." His initial presentation seemed straightforward—relationship problems and communication difficulties. But the integration formulation revealed a complex system (137).

Layer 1: Presenting Concerns Robert described feeling "disconnected" from his wife and children, working excessive hours, and experiencing anxiety during family conflicts. His wife reported feeling like she was "married to a stranger" who disappeared emotionally whenever situations became challenging.

Layer 2: Schema Architecture Assessment revealed strong Emotional Inhibition and Subjugation schemas rooted in childhood with an alcoholic father and overwhelmed mother. His Unrelenting Standards schema drove perfectionism at work. His Mistrust/Abuse schema created hypervigilance in relationships.

Layer 3: Trauma and Memory Networks Robert's trauma history included emotional neglect, parentification (caring for younger siblings while parents struggled), and witnessing domestic violence. Key schema-maintaining memories included being told "big boys don't cry" at age six and being punished for expressing anger at age ten.

Layer 4: Mode and Parts Constellation His internal system included:

- **Detached Protector Mode**: Primary coping strategy that created emotional distance during stress
- **Vulnerable Child Mode**: Carried unexpressed sadness and fear from childhood
- **Punitive Parent Mode**: Criticized any emotional expression as weakness
- **Compliant Surrenderer Mode**: Automatically agreed to avoid conflict
- **Healthy Adult Mode**: Significantly underdeveloped

Layer 5: Somatic Patterns Robert's body told the story his words couldn't express. Chronic tension in jaw and shoulders reflected emotional control. Shallow breathing prevented full emotional experience. His posture remained rigid even in safe environments.

Layer 6: Strengths and Resources Despite his challenges, Robert showed significant strengths: high intelligence, strong work ethic, deep love for his family (though expressed through providing rather than emotional connection), and motivation for change. His wife's ultimatum, while painful, represented an opportunity for growth.

Integration Formulation Summary Robert's emotional unavailability represented a protective system developed in childhood to survive in an unsafe emotional environment. His Detached Protector mode, while adaptive during childhood chaos, now prevented the intimacy his family needed. His schemas created a feedback loop where emotional expression felt dangerous, leading to withdrawal, which created the very rejection he feared.

The formulation suggested that healing required helping Robert's protective parts understand that his current family was safe for emotional expression. EMDR could process childhood memories that taught him emotions were dangerous. Somatic work could help him reconnect with his body's emotional wisdom. Schema mode work could strengthen his Healthy Adult and help his protective parts find updated roles.

Case Example: Linda's Complex Presentation

Linda, a 29-year-old social worker, presented with what initially appeared to be straightforward depression and anxiety. But her integration formulation revealed a trauma-informed constellation requiring careful treatment planning (138).

Layer 1: Presenting Concerns Linda reported chronic fatigue, relationship difficulties, and feeling "empty inside." She struggled with boundaries at work, often staying late to help clients while neglecting her own needs. Her romantic relationships followed a pattern of intense connection followed by withdrawal.

Layer 2: Schema Architecture Assessment revealed primary schemas of Self-Sacrifice, Emotional Deprivation, Abandonment, and Defectiveness. These patterns created a cycle where she gave excessively to others while feeling empty and unworthy of receiving care herself.

Layer 3: Trauma and Memory Networks Linda's history included childhood emotional neglect, parentification with a depressed mother, and sexual abuse by a family friend at age twelve. The abuse had never been processed or disclosed. Recent relationship difficulties were triggering memories of betrayal and powerlessness.

Layer 4: Mode and Parts Constellation Her internal system was complex:

- **Vulnerable Child Mode**: Carried pain from neglect and abuse
- **Angry Child Mode**: Held rage about unmet needs and violation
- **Self-Sacrifice Mode**: Compulsively cared for others while ignoring own needs
- **Detached Protector Mode**: Created emotional numbing during overwhelm
- **Punitive Parent Mode**: Attacked her for having needs or setting boundaries

Layer 5: Somatic Patterns Linda's body reflected her psychological fragmentation. She experienced chronic pain without clear medical cause, frequent illness suggesting immune system compromise, and dissociative episodes during stress. Her breathing remained shallow and her posture collapsed, as if trying to make herself invisible.

Layer 6: Strengths and Resources Despite her struggles, Linda showed remarkable resilience and compassion. Her work as a social worker demonstrated her capacity for empathy and helping others. She had two close friendships that provided some support. Her intelligence and introspection suggested good therapy readiness.

Integration Formulation Summary Linda's presentation represented the long-term effects of complex developmental trauma. Her Self-Sacrifice schema developed as a survival strategy—being helpful was the only way to receive attention in her neglectful family. The sexual abuse confirmed her Defectiveness schema and taught her that her body and boundaries weren't respected.

Her current symptoms reflected an internal system organized around avoiding further harm while desperately seeking the care she never received. Her helping behaviors served multiple functions: proving her worth, avoiding abandonment, and expressing her genuine compassion while staying safely in the helper role.

Treatment planning needed to proceed carefully, with extensive stabilization before processing trauma memories. Her protective parts would need to trust the therapeutic relationship before allowing access to vulnerable aspects. Somatic work would be essential for helping her reconnect with her body safely.

Case Example: Marcus's Multicultural Integration

Marcus, a 48-year-old Puerto Rican construction supervisor, sought help for anger management after a workplace incident. His cultural background and family dynamics required careful integration into the formulation process (139).

Layer 1: Presenting Concerns Marcus described explosive anger episodes that threatened his job and marriage. He felt like "two different people"—calm and controlled most of the time, then suddenly overwhelmed by rage over minor incidents. His family was concerned about his drinking, which increased after angry episodes.

Layer 2: Schema Architecture Assessment revealed schemas that intersected with cultural factors: Mistrust/Abuse (rooted in childhood violence), Defectiveness (connected to immigration experiences), and Unrelenting Standards (influenced by cultural expectations of male providers). His Vulnerability to Harm schema was activated by perceived disrespect at work.

Layer 3: Trauma and Memory Networks Marcus's trauma included domestic violence in his family of origin, discrimination experiences after immigrating to the mainland US, and combat exposure during

79

military service. These experiences created layered trauma responses that intersected with cultural identity issues.

Layer 4: Mode and Parts Constellation His internal system reflected cultural influences:

- **Angry Child Mode**: Carried rage about injustice and disrespect
- **Vulnerable Child Mode**: Held pain about not belonging or being accepted
- **Demanding Parent Mode**: Pushed him to be strong and provide for family
- **Detached Protector Mode**: Shut down emotions to avoid appearing weak
- **Healthy Adult Mode**: Present but often overwhelmed by other modes

Layer 5: Somatic Patterns Marcus's anger had clear somatic signatures: muscle tension that built throughout the day, shallow breathing during stress, and explosive energy release during anger episodes. His cultural background included both acceptance of emotional expression and expectations of male stoicism.

Layer 6: Strengths and Resources Marcus showed significant strengths rooted in his cultural identity: strong family loyalty, excellent work ethic, leadership skills, and community connections. His spiritual beliefs provided potential resources for healing. His motivation to change was driven by love for his family.

Integration Formulation Summary Marcus's anger represented the intersection of personal trauma, cultural factors, and current stressors. His explosive episodes occurred when multiple triggers activated simultaneously: perceived disrespect (triggering discrimination memories), feeling powerless (activating childhood trauma), and pressure to remain strong (cultural expectations).

His drinking served as both self-medication and cultural coping mechanism, but was creating additional problems. Treatment needed to honor his cultural values while helping him develop updated coping strategies. His anger contained important information about injustice and boundaries that needed expression in healthier ways.

Multi-Level Assessment Framework

Integration formulation requires assessment tools that capture information across all relevant domains. Traditional diagnostic approaches often miss the complexity needed for effective integration work (140).

Cognitive Assessment:

- Schema patterns and activation triggers
- Cognitive distortions and core beliefs
- Problem-solving and coping strategies
- Intellectual and educational resources

Emotional Assessment:

- Emotional regulation capacity and patterns
- Attachment style and relationship patterns
- Mood stability and emotional range
- Historical emotional experiences and training

Somatic Assessment:

- Nervous system regulation patterns
- Body awareness and comfort levels
- Physical health and medical considerations
- Breathing, posture, and movement patterns

Spiritual Assessment:

- Meaning-making systems and values
- Connection to transcendent or spiritual experiences
- Religious or spiritual practices and communities
- Existential concerns and life purpose questions

Cultural Assessment:

- Cultural identity and acculturation level
- Family and community cultural patterns
- Language preferences and communication styles
- Cultural strengths and challenges in treatment

Social Assessment:

- Support systems and relationship quality
- Work and financial stability
- Community connections and social roles
- Family dynamics and relationship patterns

Creating Client-Friendly Formulations

The best formulation in the world helps nobody if your client can't understand or use it. You need skills for translating complex psychological concepts into language that makes sense to real people living real lives (141).

Use Metaphors and Analogies: Instead of saying "Your Punitive Parent mode activates when your Vulnerable Child fears abandonment," try "There's a part of you that learned to be really hard on yourself to try to prevent rejection—like having a harsh internal coach who thinks criticism will make you perfect enough that people won't leave."

Focus on Functions Rather Than Pathology: Frame patterns as attempts to solve problems rather than character defects. "Your anger makes perfect sense when we understand it as your way of trying to protect yourself from feeling powerless like you did as a child."

Connect Past to Present: Help clients understand how their patterns developed and why they made sense at the time. "The strategies you learned as a kid to survive in your family are still trying to protect you, but they're not needed in the same way now."

Emphasize Choice and Agency: Frame formulation as providing options rather than deterministic explanations. "Now that we understand how these patterns work, you have choices about how to respond when they get triggered."

Collaborative Treatment Planning

Integration treatment planning requires genuine collaboration with clients as partners in their healing process. This isn't just good therapy—it's practical necessity for complex integration work (142).

Shared Decision-Making Process:

1. **Present the formulation** in understandable language
2. **Gather client feedback** and corrections to the formulation
3. **Identify priority targets** based on client values and goals
4. **Discuss modality options** and explain rationales for different approaches
5. **Create timeline and milestones** with flexibility for adjustments
6. **Establish collaboration agreements** about roles and responsibilities

Priority Setting Framework: Help clients identify what matters most to them right now. Safety issues take priority, but within safety parameters, let client values guide the focus. Someone might prioritize work functioning over relationship issues, or vice versa.

Modality Education: Clients need enough understanding of different approaches to participate meaningfully in treatment planning. Explain how EMDR, schema work, somatic approaches, and parts work might help their specific situation.

Cultural Integration in Planning: Include cultural factors explicitly in treatment planning. How do cultural values intersect with treatment goals? What cultural resources can support healing? How can treatment honor cultural identity while promoting growth?

Visual Mapping Systems

Many clients understand their internal world better through visual representations than verbal descriptions. Visual mapping tools can make complex formulations accessible and memorable (143).

Schema Mapping Diagrams: Create visual representations of how different schemas interact and trigger each other. Use colors, shapes, or symbols that resonate with your client's preferred learning style.

Parts and Modes Maps: Draw the client's internal system showing different parts or modes and their relationships. Include protective functions and communication patterns between parts.

Trauma Timeline Graphics: Create visual timelines that show how traumatic experiences connect to current patterns. Help clients see themes and connections across their life story.

Nervous System Maps: Illustrate how their nervous system responds to different triggers and what regulation looks like for them specifically. Include their personal warning signs and recovery strategies.

Resource and Strength Inventories: Create visual representations of their existing resources, support systems, and positive qualities. This provides balance to problem-focused assessment.

Target Hierarchy Development

Integration work can feel overwhelming without clear priorities. Target hierarchy development helps organize the work while maintaining flexibility for client needs and clinical judgment (144).

Safety and Stabilization Targets:

- Crisis management and safety planning
- Basic self-care and daily functioning
- Nervous system regulation skills

- Support system strengthening

Processing and Integration Targets:

- Schema-maintaining trauma memories
- Mode integration and internal communication
- Somatic pattern transformation
- Relationship pattern changes

Application and Maintenance Targets:

- Daily life skill implementation
- Relationship and work integration
- Relapse prevention and maintenance
- Ongoing growth and development

Flexibility in Target Selection: Maintain responsiveness to client needs and emerging priorities. Sometimes a crisis requires shifting focus. Sometimes unexpected breakthroughs create new opportunities for growth.

Managing Formulation Complexity

Integration formulations can become so complex that they lose clinical utility. You need strategies for managing complexity while maintaining nuance (145).

Layered Disclosure: Present formulation information gradually rather than overwhelming clients with everything at once. Start with basic patterns and add complexity as they're ready to integrate more information.

Focus and Prioritization: Identify the most important patterns for current functioning rather than trying to address everything simultaneously. You can always add complexity later as foundational work progresses.

Regular Review and Updates: Formulations should evolve as you learn more about your client and as they grow and change. Schedule regular formulation review sessions to update understanding and adjust treatment plans.

Consultation and Supervision: Complex formulations benefit from outside perspectives. Use consultation to ensure you're not missing important information or getting lost in unnecessary complexity.

Documentation and Communication

Integration formulations need documentation systems that support clinical work while meeting professional and legal requirements (146).

Clinical Documentation Requirements:

- Clear diagnostic impressions that support integration rationale
- Treatment plans that specify modalities and rationales
- Progress notes that track changes across multiple domains
- Safety assessments that address all relevant risk factors

Communication with Other Providers: When working with treatment teams, you need skills for communicating integration formulations to professionals who may not understand multi-modal approaches. Focus on functional improvements and evidence-based rationales.

Insurance and Authorization Considerations: Insurance systems often don't recognize integration approaches. Learn to present integration work within frameworks that insurance understands while maintaining clinical integrity.

Building Integration Communities

Integration formulation represents a different way of thinking about human psychological experience—one that honors complexity while maintaining clinical utility. As more therapists develop these skills, we're building communities of practice that can support and advance this approach (147).

Your formulation work contributes to the larger project of understanding how human beings heal and grow. Each client teaches us something new about the intersection of trauma, schemas, body wisdom, and resilience. This knowledge belongs not just to individual therapeutic relationships but to the broader community of healers working toward more effective and humane approaches to psychological distress.

The formulations you create today become the foundation for tomorrow's innovations in integration work. You're not just helping individual clients—you're participating in the evolution of therapeutic practice itself.

Essential Principles for Practice

Integration formulation requires shifting from symptom-focused thinking to pattern-based understanding of human experience. Your formulations become roadmaps for healing that honor both the complexity of psychological distress and the innate human capacity for growth and change. The next chapter examines how these principles apply to the most challenging presentations—complex cases that test our integration skills and demand our most sophisticated clinical thinking.

Key Learning Principles

- Multi-layered formulation captures the full complexity of human psychological experience across cognitive, emotional, somatic, and cultural domains
- Client-friendly explanations require translating professional concepts into accessible language that empowers rather than pathologizes
- Collaborative treatment planning transforms clients from passive recipients to active partners in their healing process

- Visual mapping systems help clients understand their internal world and track progress across multiple domains
- Target hierarchy development organizes complex integration work while maintaining flexibility for emerging needs and opportunities
- Regular formulation review and updates ensure that treatment remains responsive to client growth and changing circumstances

Chapter 8: Managing Complex Cases

Complex cases find their way to integration practitioners like iron filings to a magnet. You know the clients I mean—the ones who've been through multiple therapists, carry several diagnoses, and present with symptoms that seem to resist standard treatments (148). These aren't failures of previous therapy; they're human beings whose psychological organization requires the sophistication that only integration approaches can provide.

Sarah walks into your office carrying a file thick with previous treatment attempts. Diagnoses include Major Depression, PTSD, Borderline Personality Disorder, and "rule out" Dissociative Identity Disorder. She's tried individual therapy, group therapy, medication trials, and intensive outpatient programs. Each helped somewhat, but nothing created lasting change. Her presentation includes mood instability, relationship chaos, self-harm behaviors, and dissociative episodes that leave her feeling fragmented and hopeless.

Complex cases challenge everything you think you know about therapy. They demand clinical sophistication, emotional resilience, and systematic approaches that can hold multiple levels of intervention simultaneously. This chapter provides frameworks for managing complexity without losing your therapeutic center or compromising client safety (149).

Understanding Complex Presentations

Complex cases aren't just complicated cases. Complexity emerges from specific factors that create multiplicative rather than additive treatment challenges (150).

Multiple Trauma Types: Complex clients often present with layered trauma experiences across development. Childhood abuse, neglect, attachment disruption, medical trauma, and adult retraumatization create interconnected networks of dysregulation that resist single-modality approaches.

Severe Schema Consolidation: Instead of one or two problematic schemas, complex clients often score high across multiple schema domains. Their early maladaptive schemas reinforce each other, creating rigid personality organization that feels impossible to change.

Dissociative Processes: Many complex clients use dissociation as a primary coping mechanism. This creates therapeutic challenges because parts of their experience remain disconnected from conscious processing and integration.

Multiple Diagnoses and Symptom Clusters: Complex clients rarely fit neat diagnostic categories. They present with symptoms that cross traditional boundaries—mood disorders, anxiety, trauma responses, personality features, and sometimes psychotic symptoms.

Life Instability: Chronic relationship difficulties, employment problems, financial instability, and ongoing life crises create environments that maintain psychological dysregulation and interfere with consistent therapeutic work.

Treatment History and Resistance: Previous negative therapy experiences can create treatment resistance and hypervigilance about therapeutic relationships. Clients may simultaneously desperately want help while protecting themselves from further disappointment or harm.

Case Example: Elena's Childhood Trauma Constellation

Elena, a 34-year-old nurse, presented with what her intake summary described as "treatment-resistant depression with trauma features." Her complexity became apparent during assessment when standard approaches failed to capture her internal experience (151).

Initial Presentation: Elena reported chronic depression, anxiety, relationship instability, and work difficulties. She'd been in therapy on and off for fifteen years with minimal lasting improvement. Her current crisis involved a breakup that triggered suicidal ideation and self-harm behaviors.

Trauma History Discovery: Initial trauma screening revealed childhood sexual abuse, but deeper assessment uncovered a constellation of developmental trauma:

- Sexual abuse by stepfather from ages 6-12
- Emotional neglect by overwhelmed mother
- Medical trauma from multiple hospitalizations for chronic illness
- Bullying at school with no family support
- Parentification caring for younger siblings
- Witnessing domestic violence between mother and stepfather

Schema Consolidation: Elena scored in clinical ranges on 14 of 18 early maladaptive schemas. Her schema patterns reinforced each other in ways that created rigid personality organization. Her Abandonment and Defectiveness schemas made relationships feel threatening. Her Self-Sacrifice schema kept her in helper roles while her Emotional Deprivation schema left her feeling empty.

Dissociative Presentation: Elena described feeling like "different people" in different situations. Assessment revealed:

- Amnesia for parts of her childhood and some recent events
- Identity confusion and sense of internal multiplicity
- Depersonalization and derealization during stress
- Time loss and finding evidence of activities she couldn't recall
- Different "parts" with distinct preferences, memories, and ways of being

Internal System Complexity: Schema mode and IFS assessment revealed a complex internal system:

- Multiple Child parts holding different aspects of trauma
- Rigid Protector parts that controlled access to memories and emotions
- Punitive parts that maintained safety through self-attack
- Host part that managed daily functioning while staying disconnected from internal experience

Treatment Planning Challenges: Elena's complexity required treatment planning that could address:

- Severe trauma history across multiple developmental periods
- Dissociative processes that fragmented her experience
- Complex schema patterns that maintained suffering
- Suicidal ideation and self-harm behaviors
- Life instability and relationship chaos
- Previous treatment failures and therapeutic mistrust

Case Example: Michael's Personality Disorder Integration

Michael, a 41-year-old attorney, sought treatment after his law firm mandated therapy following complaints about his interpersonal behavior. His presentation illustrated how personality disorder features require specialized integration approaches (152).

Clinical Presentation: Michael met criteria for Narcissistic Personality Disorder with borderline features. He alternated between grandiose self-presentation and crushing shame, maintained few genuine relationships, and struggled with empathy despite high intellectual functioning.

Developmental History: Michael's childhood included:

- Narcissistic mother who alternated between idealization and devaluation
- Absent father who provided financial support but no emotional connection
- Achievement-focused family culture where worth depended on performance
- Early academic and athletic success that reinforced grandiose self-image
- Emotional neglect disguised as high expectations

Schema and Mode Constellation: Michael's internal organization included:

- **Grandiose schemas**: Entitlement and superiority beliefs that masked deep shame
- **Vulnerability schemas**: Defectiveness and Abandonment fears hidden beneath grandiose presentation
- **Grandiose Self mode**: Inflated, superior presentation used for protection
- **Vulnerable Child mode**: Carried shame and fear of being ordinary or flawed
- **Punitive Parent mode**: Harsh internal critic that prevented vulnerability
- **Detached Self-Soother mode**: Used work achievement and material success for regulation

Interpersonal Patterns: Michael's relationships followed predictable cycles:

- Initial idealization of people who could enhance his image
- Gradual devaluation when others failed to meet unrealistic expectations
- Explosive anger when his grandiose self-image was threatened
- Abandonment by others who couldn't tolerate his interpersonal style
- Confirmation of his belief that people were unreliable and disappointing

Treatment Resistance: Michael's personality organization created specific treatment challenges:

- Difficulty acknowledging problems without catastrophic shame
- Tendency to idealize or devalue the therapist
- Resistance to vulnerability required for meaningful change
- Use of intellectual understanding to avoid emotional processing
- Grandiose expectations about therapy progress and outcomes

Integration Approach: Treatment required careful attention to:

- Building therapeutic alliance that could withstand his idealization/devaluation patterns
- Addressing narcissistic vulnerability without triggering shame-based collapse
- Integrating grandiose and vulnerable aspects of his personality
- Processing childhood experiences that created his defensive organization
- Developing genuine empathy and interpersonal skills

Case Example: Lisa's Dual Diagnosis Challenge

Lisa, a 29-year-old artist, presented with co-occurring PTSD and substance use disorder. Her case illustrated the complexity of dual diagnosis presentations that require integrated treatment approaches (153).

Presenting Problems: Lisa sought help for cocaine addiction that was threatening her career and relationships. Initial assessment revealed that her substance use was closely connected to trauma symptoms and schema patterns that hadn't been addressed in previous addiction treatment.

Trauma and Addiction Intersection: Lisa's substance use served multiple functions:

- Self-medication for PTSD symptoms (flashbacks, nightmares, hypervigilance)
- Emotional numbing to manage overwhelming feelings
- Social lubrication to counter social anxiety and shame
- Energy management for creative work when depression interfered
- Punishment and self-harm expression of guilt and shame

Schema-Addiction Connections: Her early maladaptive schemas both contributed to addiction risk and were maintained by substance use:

- **Defectiveness schema**: Drove shame that fueled both using and hiding her addiction
- **Emotional Deprivation schema**: Led to using drugs for comfort and connection
- **Self-Sacrifice schema**: Prevented her from prioritizing her own recovery needs
- **Vulnerability to Harm schema**: Created anxiety that drugs temporarily relieved

Complex Trauma History: Lisa's trauma included:

- Childhood sexual abuse by family friend
- Emotional neglect in chaotic household with addicted parents
- Adult sexual assault that triggered return to heavy drug use
- Multiple losses and betrayals that reinforced attachment fears

Treatment Planning Complexity: Lisa's dual diagnosis required integration of:

- Trauma processing that accounted for addiction vulnerability
- Addiction treatment that addressed underlying trauma and schema patterns
- Schema work that supported both trauma recovery and addiction recovery
- Somatic approaches that provided regulation alternatives to substance use
- Relapse prevention that addressed trauma triggers alongside addiction triggers

Sequential vs. Integrated Treatment: Previous treatment had attempted to address her addiction and trauma separately, leading to poor outcomes. Integration required simultaneous attention to both conditions, recognizing their interconnected nature.

Titrated Integration for Fragile Clients

Complex clients often have limited capacity for traditional therapy intensity. Titrated integration provides smaller doses of therapeutic work with more stabilization time between sessions (154).

Pacing Principles:

- **Stabilization First**: Extensive preparation before any processing work
- **Smaller Doses**: Brief periods of activation with longer integration time
- **Frequent Check-ins**: More assessment of client capacity and safety
- **Flexible Scheduling**: Adjusting session frequency based on client stability
- **Multiple Resources**: Building extensive coping skills before challenging work

Signs That Titration Is Needed:

- Severe dissociation or fragmentation
- Active suicidal ideation or self-harm behaviors
- Substance use or other addictive behaviors
- Severe life instability or ongoing trauma exposure
- Previous negative reactions to therapy
- Limited support systems or social isolation

Titration Strategies:

- Extend stabilization phase from weeks to months
- Use shorter sessions (30-45 minutes) when needed
- Focus on present-moment regulation before historical processing
- Build extensive safety planning and coping resources
- Include family or support system in treatment when appropriate
- Coordinate with other providers (psychiatry, medical, case management)

Parallel Processing for Complex Systems

Some complex clients require parallel processing approaches that work with multiple aspects of their system simultaneously rather than sequentially (155).

Parallel Processing Indications:

- Severe dissociation with distinct parts or ego states
- Multiple trauma types requiring different processing approaches
- Co-occurring conditions that reinforce each other
- Life circumstances that create ongoing stress while processing historical trauma
- Complex family or relationship dynamics that require system intervention

Coordination Strategies:

- **Internal Coordination**: Working with different parts or modes in parallel sessions
- **Provider Coordination**: Multiple therapists addressing different aspects of treatment
- **Modality Coordination**: Simultaneous use of individual, group, family, and psychiatric interventions
- **Life Domain Coordination**: Addressing work, relationships, health, and other life areas simultaneously

Example of Parallel Processing: Elena (from earlier case example) required:

- Individual trauma processing for specific abuse memories
- Parts work to improve internal communication and cooperation
- Group therapy for interpersonal skills and support
- Psychiatric care for mood stabilization
- Case management for housing and employment stability
- Family therapy to address ongoing family dysfunction

Team Approaches for High-Risk Cases

Complex cases often require treatment teams rather than individual therapists working in isolation. Team approaches provide safety, expertise, and support for both clients and providers (156).

Team Composition Options:

- **Core Team**: Primary therapist, psychiatrist, case manager
- **Extended Team**: Group therapist, family therapist, substance abuse counselor
- **Specialist Consultants**: Trauma specialists, personality disorder experts, cultural consultants
- **Support Network**: Medical providers, legal advocates, spiritual care providers

Communication and Coordination:

- Regular team meetings to coordinate care and share information
- Clear communication protocols and documentation systems
- Defined roles and responsibilities for each team member
- Crisis management plans that specify who does what when
- Client involvement in team decisions and treatment planning

Benefits of Team Approaches:

- Shared responsibility for complex decision-making
- Multiple perspectives on treatment planning and progress
- Safety net for crisis situations and provider burnout
- Specialized expertise for specific aspects of treatment
- Support and consultation for primary therapist

Crisis Management in Integration Work

Complex clients often experience crises that require immediate intervention while maintaining integration principles (157).

Crisis Types in Complex Cases:

- **Suicidal Crises**: Active suicidal ideation or plans requiring immediate safety intervention
- **Dissociative Crises**: Severe fragmentation or loss of orientation requiring grounding
- **Substance Use Crises**: Relapse or escalation requiring addiction intervention
- **Relationship Crises**: Domestic violence, custody issues, or other interpersonal emergencies
- **Life Circumstances**: Housing, employment, legal, or financial crises

Integration-Informed Crisis Intervention:

- **Schema-Informed Safety Planning**: Understanding how schemas influence suicidal thinking
- **Parts-Based Crisis Work**: Accessing internal resources and protective parts during crisis
- **Somatic Crisis Intervention**: Using nervous system regulation during acute distress
- **Trauma-Informed Crisis Response**: Avoiding retraumatization during crisis intervention

Crisis Prevention Strategies:

- **Early Warning Systems**: Teaching clients to recognize escalation patterns
- **Crisis Resource Planning**: Predetermined strategies for managing different types of crises
- **Support System Activation**: Clear plans for when and how to contact support people
- **Professional Backup**: 24-hour crisis coverage and clear escalation procedures

Resistance in Complex Cases

Treatment resistance in complex cases often represents protective functions rather than opposition to change. Understanding resistance as information rather than obstacle transforms therapeutic approach (158).

Sources of Resistance:

- **Protective Parts**: Internal protectors trying to prevent retraumatization
- **Secondary Gains**: Symptoms that serve important functions in client's life
- **System Resistance**: Family or social systems that maintain dysfunction
- **Cultural Conflicts**: Treatment approaches that conflict with cultural values
- **Previous Trauma**: Therapy relationships that replicate past betrayals or violations

Working with Resistance:

- **Curiosity Rather Than Confrontation**: Exploring resistance as valuable information
- **Permission-Seeking**: Asking protective parts for consent before challenging work
- **Function Analysis**: Understanding what symptoms or behaviors accomplish
- **Cultural Consultation**: Adapting approaches to honor cultural values
- **Alliance Repair**: Addressing therapeutic ruptures quickly and directly

Documentation and Risk Management

Complex cases require enhanced documentation to manage risk and ensure continuity of care (159).

Documentation Requirements:

- **Detailed Risk Assessments**: Regular evaluation of suicide, self-harm, and violence risk
- **Treatment Rationale**: Clear explanation of integration approach and modality selection
- **Crisis Plans**: Documented safety planning and emergency procedures
- **Team Communication**: Records of consultation and coordination with other providers
- **Progress Monitoring**: Regular assessment of functioning across multiple domains

Risk Management Strategies:

- **Consultation**: Regular supervision or consultation for complex cases
- **Insurance Considerations**: Documentation that supports medical necessity
- **Legal Protections**: Understanding duty to warn and other legal obligations
- **Scope of Practice**: Staying within competence areas and referring when appropriate
- **Self-Care**: Managing therapist stress and burnout with demanding cases

Building Resilience in Complex Treatment

Working with complex cases requires resilience-building strategies for both clients and therapists. The work can be intense and demanding, requiring sustainable approaches (160).

Client Resilience Building:

- **Strength Identification**: Regular focus on client capacities and resources
- **Meaning-Making**: Helping clients find purpose and significance in their struggle
- **Connection Building**: Developing relationships that provide ongoing support

- **Skill Development**: Teaching concrete tools for managing symptoms and stress
- **Hope Restoration**: Maintaining realistic optimism about possibility for change

Therapist Resilience Strategies:

- **Regular Supervision**: Ongoing consultation and support for clinical decision-making
- **Personal Therapy**: Addressing therapist's own trauma and attachment issues
- **Professional Development**: Continuing education and skill building
- **Work-Life Balance**: Maintaining boundaries and outside interests
- **Peer Support**: Connection with colleagues who understand complex case challenges

The Rewards of Complex Work

Working with complex cases tests every skill you possess while teaching you things no textbook can convey. These clients become your greatest teachers, showing you the remarkable resilience of the human spirit and the healing power of relationship and understanding (161).

Success with complex cases doesn't look like traditional therapy outcomes. Progress appears in smaller increments—a client who calls instead of cutting, someone who recognizes a trigger before it overwhelms them, a person who maintains employment for six months instead of six weeks. These seemingly small changes represent monumental shifts in internal organization and functioning.

Complex clients remind you why you became a therapist in the first place. They challenge you to grow, to develop new skills, and to maintain hope in the face of seemingly impossible circumstances. They teach you that healing is possible even in the most difficult situations, and that integration approaches offer tools powerful enough to address the full spectrum of human suffering.

Preparing for Mastery

Complex case management represents the advanced practice of integration work. These skills prepare you for the ongoing challenge of developing competence across multiple modalities while maintaining the ethical standards and professional development necessary for safe and effective practice. Our next chapter examines the training and supervision requirements for integration practitioners.

Key Mastery Elements

- Complex cases require titrated approaches that provide smaller doses of intervention with more stabilization time
- Parallel processing allows simultaneous work with multiple aspects of complex presentations rather than sequential treatment
- Team approaches provide safety nets and specialized expertise necessary for high-risk complex cases
- Crisis management in integration work requires schema-informed, parts-based, and trauma-informed intervention strategies
- Treatment resistance often represents protective functions that provide valuable information about client needs and safety concerns
- Documentation and risk management become increasingly important with complex presentations requiring clear rationales and safety planning

Chapter 9: Training and Supervision Considerations

The path to integration competence isn't found in weekend workshops or online certificates—it requires systematic skill development across multiple modalities and years of supervised practice (162). You can't fake your way through integration work. Clients with complex presentations will quickly expose gaps in your training and challenge areas where your understanding remains superficial.

Think about Maria, sitting across from you describing childhood trauma while her Punitive Parent mode attacks her for "being dramatic," her body shows signs of hyperarousal, and her protective parts resist the vulnerability required for healing. This moment demands competence in trauma processing, schema mode work, somatic awareness, and parts-based intervention. You need more than intellectual understanding—you need embodied skills that allow you to respond effectively while maintaining safety (163).

This chapter examines the training pathways, supervision models, and ongoing development requirements for integration practitioners. The field lacks standardized training protocols, so you'll need to create your own development plan while navigating the complex landscape of certification requirements across different modalities.

Understanding Certification Pathways

Each modality that contributes to integration work has its own training requirements and certification processes. Understanding these pathways helps you plan a systematic approach to skill development (164).

Schema Therapy Certification (ISST): The International Society of Schema Therapy offers a structured certification pathway that includes:

- **Level 1 Training**: Basic concepts, assessment, and simple interventions (24 hours)
- **Level 2 Training**: Advanced techniques, complex cases, and supervision (32 hours)
- **Individual Certification Process**: Supervised practice, case presentations, and examination
- **Trainer Certification**: Advanced pathway for teaching schema therapy
- **Supervisor Certification**: Specialized training for providing schema therapy supervision

EMDR Certification (EMDRIA): The EMDR International Association provides certification through approved training programs:

- **Basic Training**: Two weekend workshops covering standard protocols (50 hours)
- **Practicum Requirements**: 50 hours of EMDR therapy with 20 different clients
- **Consultation Hours**: 20 hours of individual consultation with EMDR consultant
- **Continuing Education**: Ongoing training requirements for maintaining certification
- **Consultant Training**: Advanced pathway for providing EMDR consultation

IFS Certification: The Center for Self Leadership offers Internal Family Systems training:

- **Level 1 Training**: Basic concepts and self-leadership development (48 hours)
- **Level 2 Training**: Advanced techniques and consultation training (32 hours)
- **Level 3 Training**: Consultant certification and complex case management (32 hours)
- **Personal IFS Work**: Required therapy experience using IFS approach

- **Ongoing Training**: Annual requirements for maintaining certification

Somatic Therapy Training: Multiple organizations offer somatic therapy training with varying requirements:

- **Somatic Experiencing**: Three-year certification program through SETI
- **Sensorimotor Psychotherapy**: Multi-year training through Sensorimotor Psychotherapy Institute
- **Body-Based Therapies**: Various approaches through different training institutes
- **Integration Focus**: Specialized programs combining somatic and talk therapy approaches

Case Example: Dr. Jennifer's Training Journey

Dr. Jennifer Martinez, a licensed clinical psychologist with ten years of experience, decided to develop integration competence after recognizing limitations in her traditional CBT training. Her journey illustrates both opportunities and challenges in building integration skills (165).

Starting Point Assessment: Jennifer began with strong foundational skills:

- Licensed psychologist with solid clinical experience
- Training in cognitive-behavioral approaches
- Experience with trauma populations
- Strong therapeutic relationship skills
- Previous supervision experience

Year One: Foundation Building: Jennifer started with Schema Therapy training because it provided a framework for understanding her existing CBT skills within a broader context. She completed Level 1 training and began implementing basic schema concepts with existing clients.

Challenges Encountered:

- Intellectual understanding without embodied experience
- Difficulty recognizing schema modes in real-time
- Tendency to rush to interventions without adequate assessment
- Limited understanding of how to pace schema work safely

Supervision and Practice Development: Jennifer arranged monthly consultation with a schema therapy trainer and began keeping detailed notes about client responses to schema interventions. She practiced schema assessment with all new clients to build pattern recognition skills.

Year Two: EMDR Training: Jennifer completed EMDR basic training and began the consultation process. She discovered that combining EMDR with schema work created powerful results but also increased complexity.

Integration Challenges:

- Knowing when to use EMDR versus schema interventions
- Managing client reactions when modalities triggered different responses
- Maintaining coherent treatment plans across modalities
- Building confidence with unfamiliar techniques

Year Three: IFS and Somatic Training: Jennifer added IFS Level 1 training and a year-long somatic therapy program. She began to understand how all four modalities could work together systematically.

Personal Development Requirements: Each training program required Jennifer to experience the modalities personally:

- Schema therapy for understanding her own patterns
- EMDR processing for personal trauma history
- IFS work for internal system development

- Somatic therapy for body awareness and regulation

Year Four: Integration Practice: Jennifer developed confidence in combining modalities and began accepting more complex referrals. She noticed significant improvements in client outcomes and her own therapeutic satisfaction.

Ongoing Development: Jennifer continues attending advanced workshops, maintains consultation relationships, and participates in professional organizations. She now provides consultation to other therapists beginning integration training.

Case Example: Robert's Supervision Challenge

Robert Thompson, a licensed clinical social worker, attempted to develop integration skills without adequate supervision and encountered significant difficulties (166).

Background and Training: Robert had fifteen years of experience in community mental health and completed weekend workshops in Schema Therapy and EMDR. He believed this training was sufficient to begin integration work.

Early Implementation Problems:

- Client became increasingly unstable after Robert attempted schema mode work
- EMDR processing session resulted in severe dissociation that Robert couldn't manage
- Robert felt overwhelmed and unprepared for client reactions
- Client filed complaint about feeling unsafe during sessions

Supervision Intervention: Robert's agency required him to seek specialized supervision after the complaint. His supervisor helped him understand:

- Weekend training provided introduction, not competence

- Complex clients require extensive preparation and safety planning
- Integration work demands ongoing supervision and consultation
- Personal development work supports professional competence

Remediation Plan:

- Temporary restriction from complex trauma and integration cases
- Monthly supervision focused on integration principles
- Personal therapy to address countertransference and skill gaps
- Gradual return to integration work with careful oversight

Lessons Learned: Robert's experience highlighted the importance of:

- Adequate training before implementation
- Ongoing supervision for complex cases
- Recognition of competence limits and scope of practice
- Systematic skill development rather than piecemeal training

Case Example: Dr. Sarah's Advanced Practice Development

Dr. Sarah Kim, a licensed psychologist, developed expertise in integration work and now provides supervision and training to other professionals (167).

Foundation Development: Sarah completed full certification in all four modalities over a six-year period:

- Schema Therapy Individual Certification (ISST)
- EMDR Certified Therapist (EMDRIA)
- IFS Level 3 Consultant
- Somatic Experiencing Practitioner (SETI)

Personal Development Component: Sarah engaged in extensive personal work:

- Two years of schema therapy addressing childhood perfectionism
- EMDR processing for medical trauma from cancer treatment
- IFS work for internal system integration
- Ongoing somatic practices for nervous system regulation

Integration Training Development: Sarah developed specialized integration training that combines all four modalities:

- Year-long training program with monthly workshops
- Supervision groups for practicing clinicians
- Consultation services for complex cases
- Research collaboration with university partners

Teaching and Supervision Philosophy: Sarah's approach emphasizes:

- Personal development as foundation for professional competence
- Systematic skill building with adequate supervision
- Integration of theory and practice through experiential learning
- Ongoing professional development and consultation

Challenges in Advanced Practice:

- Limited number of qualified supervisors for integration work
- Lack of standardized training protocols across modalities
- Insurance and liability considerations for innovative approaches
- Maintaining competence across rapidly evolving fields

Supervision Models for Integration Work

Traditional supervision models often fall short for integration work because they focus on single modalities rather than the complex decision-making required for multi-modal approaches (168).

Individual Supervision Model: One-on-one supervision with integration-trained supervisor provides:

- Personalized attention to individual learning needs
- Real-time consultation on complex cases
- Detailed feedback on technique and decision-making
- Support for personal development and professional growth

Group Supervision Model: Group supervision with integration focus offers:

- Multiple perspectives on complex cases
- Peer learning and support
- Cost-effective supervision for multiple supervisees
- Community building among integration practitioners

Consultation Team Model: Teams of specialists provide consultation across modalities:

- Schema therapy consultant for schema-related questions
- EMDR consultant for trauma processing issues
- IFS consultant for parts work challenges
- Somatic consultant for body-based interventions

Peer Consultation Model: Experienced practitioners provide mutual consultation:

- Regular meetings to discuss challenging cases
- Shared responsibility for complex treatment decisions
- Professional support and burnout prevention
- Ongoing learning and skill development

Competency Development Framework

Integration competence develops through systematic progression from basic understanding to advanced practice. Clear competency frameworks help guide development and assess readiness for independent practice (169).

Foundation Competencies:

- Understanding of human development and psychopathology
- Basic therapy skills including rapport building and safety management
- Knowledge of trauma responses and their impact on functioning
- Ethical decision-making and professional boundary management
- Cultural competence and awareness of diversity factors

Modality-Specific Competencies: Each contributing modality requires specific knowledge and skills:

- Schema Therapy: Assessment, mode work, experiential techniques
- EMDR: Standard protocols, stabilization, resource development
- IFS: Self-leadership, parts work, internal system navigation
- Somatic Approaches: Nervous system awareness, regulation techniques

Integration Competencies: Advanced skills specific to multi-modal approaches:

- Case formulation across modalities
- Treatment planning with multiple approaches
- Decision-making about modality selection and sequencing
- Managing complex therapeutic relationships
- Crisis intervention using integration principles

Supervision and Teaching Competencies: Advanced practitioners develop skills for training others:

- Supervision and consultation skills
- Training design and implementation
- Professional development and mentoring
- Research and outcome evaluation

Self-Therapy Requirements

All integration training programs require participants to experience the modalities personally. This isn't just professional development—it's essential preparation for complex clinical work (170).

Rationale for Personal Work:

- Understanding approaches from client perspective
- Identifying personal triggers and countertransference patterns
- Developing internal resources for managing difficult cases
- Building empathy and compassion for client experiences

Schema Therapy Personal Work: Therapists need awareness of their own schema patterns and how they might interfere with clinical work. Common therapist schemas include:

- Self-Sacrifice schemas that lead to overworking and boundary problems
- Unrelenting Standards that create perfectionism and self-criticism
- Emotional Inhibition that interferes with therapeutic authenticity

EMDR Personal Processing: Therapists benefit from EMDR processing to:

- Resolve personal trauma that might interfere with client work
- Understand the processing experience from client perspective
- Build comfort with emotional intensity and memory processing
- Develop personal resources for managing difficult sessions

IFS Personal Development: IFS work helps therapists:

- Develop Self-leadership and internal awareness
- Understand their own protective patterns and triggers
- Build capacity for staying present during challenging sessions

- Integrate different aspects of their personality and professional identity

Somatic Personal Practice: Body-based personal work supports therapists in:

- Developing nervous system regulation and resilience
- Understanding somatic experience and body awareness
- Building comfort with physical sensations and emotional intensity
- Maintaining personal health and preventing burnout

Continuing Education and Maintenance

Integration competence requires ongoing development because the field continues to evolve and individual skills need regular updating (171).

Annual Training Requirements: Most certification bodies require ongoing education:

- Schema Therapy: 12 hours annually for certification maintenance
- EMDR: 20 hours every two years for certified therapists
- IFS: 8 hours annually for consultant maintenance
- Somatic Approaches: Variable requirements by training organization

Advanced Training Opportunities:

- Specialized workshops for complex populations
- Integration-specific training programs
- Conference presentations and professional meetings
- Research participation and outcome studies

Self-Assessment and Skill Updates: Regular evaluation of competence and areas for growth:

- Video review of therapy sessions for skill assessment
- Client outcome tracking and treatment evaluation
- Peer feedback and consultation input
- Personal reflection and professional development planning

Ethical Considerations in Training

Integration training raises specific ethical considerations related to scope of practice, competence development, and client welfare (172).

Scope of Practice Issues:

- Understanding limits of current competence
- Knowing when to refer or seek consultation
- Maintaining certification requirements across multiple modalities
- Representing qualifications accurately to clients and colleagues

Competence Development Standards:

- Adequate training before implementation
- Ongoing supervision during skill development
- Personal development work to support professional competence
- Recognition of learning needs and areas for growth

Client Welfare Considerations:

- Informed consent about training status and supervision
- Safety planning for complex cases during training
- Clear policies about emergency coverage and backup support
- Protection of client confidentiality during supervision

Building Training Infrastructure

The field needs systematic development of training infrastructure to support integration practitioners (173).

Training Program Development:

- Standardized curricula that combine multiple modalities
- Faculty development for integration training
- Clinical training sites with integration supervision
- Research programs to evaluate training effectiveness

Certification and Credentialing:

- Integration-specific certification processes
- Professional standards for integration practice
- Quality assurance for training programs
- Continuing education requirements and monitoring

Professional Organizations:

- Societies focused on integration approaches
- Professional networking and support
- Research collaboration and knowledge sharing
- Advocacy for integration recognition and reimbursement

The Future of Integration Training

Integration training continues to evolve as the field develops more sophisticated understanding of how modalities work together. Future developments may include (174):

Technology-Enhanced Training:

- Virtual reality for experiential learning
- Online platforms for supervision and consultation
- Video-based training for skill development
- Mobile apps for practice support and skill building

Research-Informed Training:

- Outcome studies to evaluate training effectiveness
- Process research to understand skill development

- Neuroscience research to inform training approaches
- Evidence-based training protocols and standards

Global Training Networks:

- International collaboration on training standards
- Cultural adaptation of training approaches
- Exchange programs for advanced training
- Multi-language training materials and resources

Sustaining Your Development Journey

Integration training represents a career-long commitment to learning and growth. The field continues to evolve, new research emerges regularly, and your own skills and understanding deepen with experience. Maintaining enthusiasm for learning while managing the demands of complex clinical work requires intention and planning (175).

Your training journey connects you to a community of practitioners committed to advancing the field of integration therapy. Each client you work with, each supervision session you attend, and each workshop you complete contributes to the broader understanding of how human beings heal and grow.

The investment you make in training prepares you for some of the most meaningful and challenging work in the field of mental health. Integration practitioners have opportunities to work with clients that other approaches cannot help, to be part of cutting-edge developments in therapy, and to contribute to the evolution of healing practices.

Professional Development Pathway

Integration training provides the foundation for ethical, effective practice, but systematic skill development must be accompanied by clear understanding of the ethical complexities that arise when combining multiple modalities. Our next chapter examines the ethical frameworks necessary for responsible integration practice.

Core Training Insights

- Integration competence requires systematic certification in multiple modalities rather than introductory workshops
- Personal development work in each modality provides essential foundation for professional competence
- Supervision models must adapt to address the complexity of multi-modal decision-making and case management
- Competency development follows predictable stages from foundation skills through advanced integration practice
- Continuing education requirements ensure ongoing skill development as the field continues to evolve
- Ethical training considerations include scope of practice, adequate preparation, and client welfare protection

Chapter 10: Ethical Issues in Integration

Integration work operates in the spaces between established modalities—territories where traditional ethical guidelines may not provide clear direction (176). You're combining approaches that weren't designed to work together, applying techniques across different theoretical frameworks, and making clinical decisions that single-modality training didn't prepare you for. This chapter examines the ethical frameworks necessary for responsible integration practice.

Consider David, a client presenting with complex PTSD who could benefit from EMDR processing combined with schema mode work and somatic regulation. Your EMDR training taught you specific protocols for trauma processing. Your schema therapy training emphasized the importance of stabilization and mode work. Your somatic training highlighted nervous system regulation. But none of your training programs addressed how to combine these approaches ethically and safely (177).

Ethical integration practice requires more than following individual modality guidelines—you need frameworks for making complex decisions about treatment planning, informed consent, cultural adaptation, and professional competence when working across multiple approaches.

Scope of Practice Boundaries

Integration work challenges traditional scope of practice boundaries because it combines techniques from different modalities that may fall under different professional regulations (178).

Understanding Professional Boundaries: Your scope of practice is defined by your professional license, state regulations, training credentials, and institutional policies. Integration doesn't expand your scope beyond these boundaries—it requires working within them while combining approaches appropriately.

License-Specific Considerations: Different mental health licenses have varying scopes related to integration work:

- **Clinical Psychologists**: Generally broad scope including assessment, therapy, and specialized interventions
- **Licensed Clinical Social Workers**: Social work scope with emphasis on person-in-environment
- **Licensed Professional Counselors**: Counseling scope that varies significantly by state
- **Marriage and Family Therapists**: Specialized scope focused on relationship and family work

Training vs. License Scope: Your training credentials don't expand your professional license scope. Having EMDR certification doesn't allow you to practice beyond your license limitations. Having schema therapy training doesn't authorize work outside your professional scope.

Institutional Policies: Many practitioners work in settings with additional scope limitations:

- Agency policies about approved treatment approaches
- Hospital or clinic protocols for specific interventions
- Insurance panels with limited reimbursement for certain approaches
- Supervision requirements for complex or specialized work

Case Example: Dr. Martinez's Scope Challenge

Dr. Martinez, a licensed professional counselor, completed training in Schema Therapy, EMDR, and somatic approaches. She began working with complex trauma clients but encountered scope of practice challenges (179).

Initial Confidence: Dr. Martinez felt well-prepared after completing certification in multiple modalities. She began accepting referrals for complex PTSD and personality disorder presentations, believing her training qualified her for this work.

Emerging Complications: Several months into integration practice, Dr. Martinez encountered difficulties:

- Client with dissociative episodes that required psychiatric consultation
- Insurance company questioned her credentials for personality disorder treatment
- Supervisor raised concerns about working beyond her training level
- Client filed complaint about feeling unsafe during intense processing work

Scope of Practice Review: Professional consultation helped Dr. Martinez understand that:

- Her LPC license didn't specifically authorize personality disorder treatment
- Integration work with complex clients required additional supervision
- State regulations prohibited certain psychological testing she was considering
- Insurance reimbursement didn't cover some integration approaches

Resolution and Learning: Dr. Martinez made several adjustments:

- Limited complex cases to those clearly within her scope
- Arranged ongoing consultation with licensed psychologist
- Developed referral relationships for psychological testing
- Created clearer informed consent about treatment limitations

Professional Growth: The experience taught Dr. Martinez important lessons about:

- Staying within scope while developing integration skills
- Importance of ongoing consultation for complex work
- Need for clear communication about scope limitations
- Value of collaboration with other professionals

Informed Consent Complexities

Integration approaches require more complex informed consent processes because clients need to understand multiple modalities and how they work together (180).

Standard Informed Consent Elements: Basic informed consent includes information about:

- Nature and goals of treatment
- Therapist qualifications and approach
- Risks and benefits of treatment
- Alternative treatment options
- Confidentiality and its limits
- Fees and business policies

Integration-Specific Additions: Integration informed consent must also address:

- Explanation of each modality being used
- Rationale for combining specific approaches
- How modalities will be sequenced and integrated
- Potential interactions between different approaches
- Therapist training and competence in each modality
- Research support for integration approaches

Cultural Considerations in Consent: Different cultural backgrounds affect understanding and acceptance of various therapeutic approaches:

- Some cultures view body-based interventions as inappropriate
- Religious or spiritual beliefs may conflict with certain techniques
- Language barriers may interfere with understanding complex explanations
- Collectivist cultures may prefer family involvement in consent decisions

Ongoing Consent Process: Integration work requires ongoing consent rather than one-time agreement:

- Regular review of treatment progress and approaches
- Consent for new modalities as treatment evolves
- Client choice about which approaches feel most helpful
- Right to discontinue specific modalities while continuing others

Case Example: Maria's Cultural Adaptation Challenge

Maria, a 45-year-old Latina client, sought help for depression and anxiety but struggled with integration approaches that conflicted with her cultural values (181).

Initial Presentation: Maria presented with symptoms of depression, anxiety, and relationship difficulties. Assessment suggested benefits from schema work, EMDR processing, and somatic approaches for trauma history.

Cultural Conflicts: Several aspects of integration treatment conflicted with Maria's cultural background:

- Somatic approaches felt inappropriate given cultural modesty values
- Individual focus conflicted with collectivist family orientation
- Emphasis on personal needs seemed selfish within cultural context
- Discussion of childhood experiences felt disrespectful to family

Adaptation Process: Maria's therapist worked collaboratively to adapt integration approaches:

- Modified somatic work to respect cultural boundaries around body awareness
- Included family perspectives in schema understanding and treatment planning

- Reframed self-care as serving family rather than selfish individual focus
- Used culturally appropriate metaphors and language for integration concepts

Successful Integration: Cultural adaptation allowed effective integration work:

- Schema work incorporated cultural values and family loyalty
- EMDR processing addressed immigration trauma within cultural context
- Somatic approaches used culturally acceptable awareness and regulation techniques
- Treatment goals aligned with cultural values while promoting healing

Learning for Practice: Maria's case highlighted importance of:

- Cultural assessment as part of integration planning
- Flexibility in adapting modalities to cultural contexts
- Collaboration with clients about cultural considerations
- Ongoing attention to cultural factors throughout treatment

Case Example: Ahmed's Religious Integration

Ahmed, a 32-year-old Muslim man, needed integration approaches that honored his religious beliefs while addressing trauma and schema patterns (182).

Religious Considerations: Ahmed's Islamic faith influenced his understanding of healing and appropriate interventions:

- Belief that healing comes ultimately from Allah required integration with therapeutic approaches
- Religious practices provided existing resources for regulation and coping
- Cultural values about gender interactions affected therapeutic relationship

- Religious community provided support system that needed integration into treatment

Adaptation Strategies: Ahmed's therapist incorporated religious perspectives:

- Schema work included Islamic concepts of fitrah (innate goodness) and spiritual development
- EMDR processing incorporated prayer and religious imagery as resources
- Somatic work respected religious guidelines about appropriate body awareness
- Treatment planning included religious advisor consultation with client permission

Integration Success: Religious integration enhanced rather than competed with therapeutic approaches:

- Religious beliefs provided framework for understanding healing process
- Islamic practices supported nervous system regulation and emotional processing
- Community support enhanced treatment outcomes and maintenance
- Spiritual perspective provided meaning and hope during difficult processing work

Professional Liability Considerations

Integration work may increase professional liability exposure because you're working outside established single-modality protocols and combining approaches in innovative ways (183).

Liability Risk Factors:

- Working beyond documented competence areas
- Combining modalities without adequate training
- Poor documentation of integration rationale

- Inadequate informed consent for complex approaches
- Boundary violations during intense integration work

Risk Management Strategies:

- Maintain extensive documentation of training and competence
- Obtain adequate professional liability insurance
- Use clear informed consent processes
- Maintain ongoing supervision or consultation
- Stay within scope of practice and documented competence

Insurance Considerations: Professional liability insurance may not automatically cover integration approaches:

- Review policies for coverage of specific modalities
- Notify insurance company about integration practice
- Document training and certification in all modalities used
- Maintain careful records of supervision and consultation

Documentation Requirements: Integration work requires enhanced documentation:

- Clear rationale for modality selection and combination
- Progress notes that address all modalities being used
- Safety assessments and crisis planning
- Supervision notes and consultation records
- Training certificates and continuing education records

Cultural Competence in Integration

Integration approaches must be adapted to work effectively across different cultural contexts while maintaining therapeutic integrity (184).

Cultural Assessment Framework: Effective cultural integration requires systematic assessment of:

- Cultural identity and acculturation level

- Language preferences and communication styles
- Religious and spiritual beliefs and practices
- Family and community cultural patterns
- Previous experiences with mental health treatment
- Cultural strengths and resources available

Modality Adaptation Considerations: Different modalities require different cultural adaptations:

- **Schema Therapy**: Adapting schema concepts to cultural values and family structures
- **EMDR**: Incorporating cultural imagery and resources into processing
- **IFS**: Adapting parts language to cultural concepts of self and identity
- **Somatic Approaches**: Respecting cultural boundaries around body awareness and touch

Language and Communication: Cultural competence includes attention to language factors:

- Working with interpreters when needed
- Using culturally appropriate metaphors and examples
- Adapting integration concepts to client's language preferences
- Understanding cultural communication styles and nonverbal patterns

Ethical Decision-Making Framework

Integration work requires systematic approaches to ethical decision-making because standard guidelines may not address complex multi-modal situations (185).

Decision-Making Process:

1. **Identify the ethical issue** and stakeholders involved
2. **Gather relevant information** about client needs, cultural factors, and treatment options

3. **Consider ethical principles** including autonomy, beneficence, non-maleficence, and justice
4. **Consult relevant guidelines** from professional organizations and licensing boards
5. **Seek consultation** with supervisors, colleagues, or ethics committees
6. **Consider alternatives** and their potential consequences
7. **Make decision** based on client welfare and ethical principles
8. **Monitor outcomes** and be prepared to adjust if needed

Ethical Principles in Integration:

- **Autonomy**: Respecting client choice about modalities and treatment approaches
- **Beneficence**: Using integration to maximize therapeutic benefit
- **Non-maleficence**: Avoiding harm through inadequate training or inappropriate combinations
- **Justice**: Ensuring fair access to integration approaches regardless of cultural background

Common Ethical Dilemmas:

- Balancing client preferences with clinical judgment about appropriate modalities
- Managing dual relationships when providing supervision and therapy
- Addressing cultural conflicts with evidence-based treatment approaches
- Handling insurance limitations that interfere with optimal integration treatment

Consultation and Collaboration

Ethical integration practice requires ongoing consultation and collaboration with other professionals (186).

Supervision Requirements:

- Regular supervision for complex integration cases
- Consultation with specialists in specific modalities
- Peer consultation groups for integration practitioners
- Emergency consultation availability for crisis situations

Collaborative Relationships:

- Psychiatrists for medication management and complex cases
- Medical professionals for health factors affecting treatment
- Cultural consultants for working across different backgrounds
- Legal consultants for complex ethical or legal issues

Documentation of Consultation:

- Records of supervision sessions and recommendations
- Consultation notes and professional advice received
- Team meeting notes and collaborative decisions
- Emergency consultation contacts and crisis planning

Building Ethical Integration Practice

Ethical integration practice develops through systematic attention to professional development, ongoing consultation, and commitment to client welfare (187).

Professional Development Plan:

- Systematic training in each modality being integrated
- Regular continuing education and skill updates
- Personal development work to address therapist factors
- Cultural competence training and ongoing education

Quality Assurance:

- Regular review of integration practices and outcomes
- Client feedback and satisfaction assessment
- Peer review and consultation input
- Ongoing supervision and professional development

Ethical Reflection:

- Regular self-assessment of ethical decision-making
- Discussion of ethical dilemmas in supervision
- Participation in professional organizations and ethics training
- Commitment to ongoing learning and improvement

The Responsibility of Innovation

Integration practitioners are pioneers in developing new approaches to healing human suffering. This innovation carries special responsibilities for ethical practice and client welfare (188).

Your work contributes to the development of treatment approaches that may help clients who haven't found relief through traditional methods. This opportunity comes with obligations to practice carefully, document thoroughly, and share knowledge responsibly.

Ethical integration practice requires humility about what you know and don't know, commitment to ongoing learning, and willingness to seek consultation when facing complex situations. The clients who seek integration approaches often have complex needs that demand your best clinical judgment and ethical reasoning.

Professional Integrity Foundation

Ethical integration practice provides the foundation for research and evidence development that advances the field while protecting client welfare. Our next chapter examines the current research base for integration approaches and opportunities for contributing to evidence-based practice development.

Fundamental Ethical Guidelines

- Scope of practice boundaries must be respected even when combining multiple modalities, with integration occurring within rather than expanding professional limits

- Informed consent processes require explanation of multiple modalities, their interaction, and ongoing consent as treatment evolves
- Cultural competence demands adaptation of integration approaches to honor client values while maintaining therapeutic effectiveness
- Professional liability management includes adequate insurance, documentation, and consultation for complex multi-modal work
- Ethical decision-making frameworks help navigate complex situations where traditional guidelines may not provide clear direction
- Ongoing consultation and collaboration ensure quality assurance and professional support for ethical integration practice

Chapter 11: Research and Evidence Base

Evidence-based practice in integration work requires understanding research that spans multiple fields while recognizing the limitations of traditional outcome studies for complex therapeutic approaches (189). You can't simply point to one randomized controlled trial and declare integration work proven—the evidence exists across studies of individual modalities, process research on therapeutic mechanisms, and emerging studies specifically examining integration approaches.

The challenge lies in translating research findings into clinical decision-making when working with real clients whose needs don't fit neatly into research protocols. Jennifer, presenting with complex PTSD, borderline personality features, and substance use history, won't find herself represented in most clinical trials. Yet research can still inform your treatment planning by helping you understand which approaches work for which aspects of complex presentations (190).

This chapter examines the current evidence base for integration approaches, identifies research gaps that need attention, and provides frameworks for applying research to clinical practice while contributing to evidence development through careful documentation and outcome tracking.

Current Evidence for Integration Approaches

The evidence base for integration work exists at multiple levels— from neuroscience research explaining why different modalities might work together to clinical trials examining specific combinations of approaches (191).

Neurobiological Research Foundation: Modern neuroscience provides the theoretical foundation for integration approaches by demonstrating that trauma and psychological distress affect multiple brain systems. Research shows that:

- Trauma impacts limbic, prefrontal, and brainstem systems differently
- Different therapeutic approaches target different neural networks
- Combining approaches may create more complete healing than single modalities
- Neuroplasticity allows for change across multiple brain systems simultaneously

Schema Therapy Research Base: Schema Therapy has substantial research support for specific populations:

- Multiple randomized controlled trials for borderline personality disorder
- Outcome studies showing superiority to treatment-as-usual for personality disorders
- Process research identifying mechanisms of change in schema interventions
- Long-term follow-up studies demonstrating maintenance of gains

EMDR Research Foundation: EMDR has extensive research support for trauma-related conditions:

- Over 30 randomized controlled trials demonstrating efficacy for PTSD
- Meta-analyses showing effectiveness comparable to other trauma treatments
- Neuroimaging studies revealing brain changes following EMDR treatment
- Research support for treating various trauma-related presentations

IFS Research Development: Internal Family Systems research is growing but less extensive:

- Pilot studies showing promise for trauma and attachment issues

- Process research examining mechanisms of Self-leadership development
- Qualitative studies documenting client experiences of parts work
- Initial outcome studies demonstrating effectiveness for various populations

Somatic Approaches Evidence: Somatic therapy research shows growing support:

- Studies of Somatic Experiencing for trauma treatment effectiveness
- Research on nervous system regulation and therapeutic outcomes
- Neuroscience research supporting body-based interventions for trauma
- Process studies examining how somatic awareness facilitates psychological change

Specific Integration Research

The most compelling evidence for integration approaches comes from studies specifically examining combined modalities rather than individual approaches (192).

The Tapia Study: EMDR-Schema Integration: The landmark study by Tapia and colleagues provided the first randomized controlled trial evidence for integration approaches. This study compared Schema Therapy alone, EMDR alone, and combined Schema Therapy-EMDR for complex PTSD presentations.

Study Design and Population:

- 90 participants with complex PTSD and comorbid conditions
- Randomized to three treatment conditions over 12 months
- Comprehensive outcome measures including trauma symptoms, personality functioning, and quality of life
- Long-term follow-up at 6 and 12 months post-treatment

Key Findings:

- Combined treatment showed superior outcomes to either approach alone
- Integration group had faster symptom reduction and better maintenance of gains
- Complex cases showed particular benefit from integration approaches
- No increase in adverse events despite treatment intensity

Clinical Implications: The Tapia study demonstrated that:

- Integration approaches can be systematically studied and shown effective
- Combined modalities may offer advantages beyond single approaches
- Complex presentations may particularly benefit from integration work
- Careful treatment planning allows safe combination of intensive modalities

Dwarshuis Integration Protocol Research: Jeff Dwarshuis's eight-step integration protocol has been examined in several smaller studies showing:

- Feasibility of systematic EMDR-Schema integration
- Improved outcomes for treatment-resistant PTSD presentations
- Client satisfaction with integration approaches
- Therapist confidence in managing complex cases using integration protocols

Case Example: Research-Informed Practice with Complex PTSD

Dr. Sarah Chen used research findings to guide integration treatment for Elena, a 32-year-old combat veteran with complex PTSD, personality disorder features, and substance use history (193).

Research-Based Assessment: Dr. Chen used research-validated instruments:

- Clinician-Administered PTSD Scale (CAPS-5) for trauma symptom assessment
- Young Schema Questionnaire for schema pattern identification
- Dissociative Experiences Scale for dissociation evaluation
- Outcome Rating Scale for ongoing progress monitoring

Evidence-Informed Treatment Planning: Based on research findings, Dr. Chen developed a phased approach:

- **Phase 1**: Stabilization using somatic regulation techniques (supported by nervous system research)
- **Phase 2**: Schema mode work to strengthen internal resources (based on schema therapy studies)
- **Phase 3**: EMDR processing of trauma memories (extensive EMDR research base)
- **Phase 4**: Integration using IFS approaches (emerging IFS research)

Treatment Implementation: Dr. Chen adapted research protocols to Elena's specific needs:

- Extended stabilization phase based on research showing importance of preparation
- Careful trauma memory sequencing following EMDR research guidelines
- Integration of schema mode work based on borderline personality disorder research
- Somatic regulation techniques supported by trauma neuroscience research

Outcome Tracking: Dr. Chen used research-validated measures to track progress:

- Monthly CAPS-5 scores showed steady symptom reduction

- Schema questionnaire scores indicated decreased schema activation
- Functional improvement measures documented daily life changes
- Client satisfaction scores remained high throughout treatment

Contribution to Evidence Base: Dr. Chen documented Elena's case systematically:

- Detailed case notes following research reporting standards
- Video recordings (with consent) for training and research purposes
- Outcome data contribution to integration research database
- Case presentation at professional conferences

Research Gaps in Integration Work

Despite growing evidence, significant gaps remain in integration research that limit clinical decision-making and treatment development (194).

Mechanism of Action Studies:

- How do different modalities interact to create therapeutic change?
- Which combinations work best for which presentations?
- What are the optimal sequencing and timing for different approaches?
- How do individual differences affect integration treatment response?

Long-Term Outcome Research:

- Do integration approaches maintain gains better than single modalities?
- What factors predict long-term success with integration treatment?

- How do clients continue to grow and change after integration therapy?
- What booster or maintenance interventions support ongoing progress?

Cultural and Diversity Research:

- How do integration approaches work across different cultural contexts?
- What adaptations are needed for specific populations?
- How do cultural factors influence treatment response and mechanisms?
- What cultural strengths can enhance integration approaches?

Training and Therapist Factors:

- What training approaches best prepare therapists for integration work?
- How do therapist characteristics influence integration treatment outcomes?
- What supervision and consultation models support effective integration practice?
- How can therapist competence in integration work be measured and maintained?

Case Example: Contributing to Research Through Practice

Dr. Michael Rodriguez developed a systematic approach to contributing research evidence through his clinical practice (195).

Practice-Based Evidence Collection: Dr. Rodriguez established systems for collecting outcome data:

- Standardized assessment battery administered at intake, mid-treatment, and termination
- Session-by-session outcome measures to track weekly progress

- Client feedback forms to capture subjective experiences
- Therapist rating scales to assess treatment process variables

Case Documentation Standards: Dr. Rodriguez used research-informed documentation:

- Detailed case formulations following integration assessment protocols
- Session notes that captured specific interventions and client responses
- Video recordings (with consent) for supervision and training purposes
- Systematic tracking of adverse events and treatment complications

Collaboration with Researchers: Dr. Rodriguez partnered with local university researchers:

- Participation in multi-site outcome studies
- Contribution of de-identified data to research databases
- Co-authorship on case study publications
- Presentation of findings at professional conferences

Quality Assurance: Dr. Rodriguez maintained research standards in practice:

- Regular supervision focused on treatment fidelity
- Peer consultation for complex cases and treatment planning
- Ongoing training to maintain competence in research-supported approaches
- Annual review of outcome data and practice patterns

Impact on Practice: Research involvement improved Dr. Rodriguez's clinical work:

- Data-driven treatment planning and modification
- Increased confidence in integration approach effectiveness

- Enhanced credibility with referral sources and insurance companies
- Professional satisfaction from contributing to field advancement

Applying Research to Clinical Decision-Making

Research application in integration work requires skills for translating study findings into clinical practice while adapting evidence to individual client needs (196).

Evidence Evaluation Framework:

1. **Study Quality Assessment**: Evaluate research design, sample characteristics, and methodology
2. **Relevance Determination**: Assess how study findings apply to your specific client population
3. **Clinical Adaptation**: Modify research protocols to fit individual client needs and circumstances
4. **Outcome Monitoring**: Track whether research-informed interventions work for specific clients
5. **Continuous Learning**: Update practice based on new research findings and clinical experience

Research-Practice Integration:

- Use research findings to inform treatment planning while maintaining clinical flexibility
- Adapt research protocols to real-world practice constraints and client preferences
- Monitor outcomes to determine if research-based interventions work for specific clients
- Contribute practice-based evidence to inform future research directions

Challenges in Research Application:

- Research samples may not represent your client population

- Research protocols may not fit practice settings or constraints
- Individual clients may not respond as research samples suggest
- Cultural and contextual factors may influence treatment response differently

Case Example: Research-Informed Cultural Adaptation

Dr. Ana Gutierrez adapted integration approaches for Latino clients based on cultural research and community input (197).

Cultural Research Review: Dr. Gutierrez examined research on:

- Latino cultural values and their influence on therapy engagement
- Traditional healing practices in Latino communities
- Research on therapy adaptations for Latino populations
- Studies of trauma and mental health in immigrant communities

Community Collaboration: Dr. Gutierrez worked with community leaders to understand:

- Cultural attitudes toward mental health treatment
- Traditional healing practices that could complement integration approaches
- Language and communication preferences
- Family and community factors affecting treatment

Adaptation Development: Based on research and community input, Dr. Gutierrez adapted integration approaches:

- **Schema Therapy**: Incorporated family loyalty and cultural values into schema understanding
- **EMDR**: Used culturally relevant imagery and resources during processing
- **IFS**: Adapted parts language to cultural concepts of self and family

- **Somatic Work**: Respected cultural boundaries while maintaining therapeutic effectiveness

Outcome Evaluation: Dr. Gutierrez tracked adapted treatment effectiveness:

- Standard outcome measures showed good treatment response
- Client satisfaction was high with culturally adapted approaches
- Treatment retention improved compared to standard approaches
- Community feedback supported continued adaptation efforts

Research Contribution: Dr. Gutierrez documented adaptation work:

- Case studies of successful cultural adaptations
- Outcome data comparing adapted versus standard approaches
- Training materials for other therapists working with Latino clients
- Conference presentations on cultural adaptation of integration work

Future Research Directions

Integration research needs to address several key areas to advance evidence-based practice and improve treatment outcomes (198).

Technology-Enhanced Research:

- Virtual reality applications for trauma processing and skill building
- Mobile apps for between-session practice and outcome monitoring
- Telehealth research on integration approaches delivery
- Artificial intelligence applications for treatment personalization

Precision Medicine Approaches:

- Research on matching specific modalities to individual client characteristics
- Biomarker research to predict treatment response and optimize approaches
- Genetic factors that influence integration treatment effectiveness
- Personalized treatment algorithms based on comprehensive assessment data

Global Research Collaboration:

- Cross-cultural research on integration approaches effectiveness
- International collaboration on training and treatment protocols
- Research on adaptation for different healthcare systems
- Global outcome databases for integration treatment research

Implementation Science Research:

- Research on how to implement integration approaches in community settings
- Training research to improve therapist competence and confidence
- Organizational factors that support or hinder integration practice
- Cost-effectiveness research on integration versus traditional approaches

Building Evidence-Based Integration Practice

Evidence-based integration practice requires balancing research findings with clinical expertise and client preferences while contributing to the growing knowledge base (199).

Personal Research Development:

- Develop skills in research evaluation and application
- Participate in outcome tracking and data collection

- Contribute to case study literature and practice-based evidence
- Collaborate with researchers on clinical questions

Professional Contribution:

- Share successful integration approaches through presentations and publications
- Mentor other therapists in evidence-based integration practice
- Participate in professional organizations advancing integration research
- Advocate for research funding and support

Clinical Excellence:

- Use research findings to inform treatment planning and intervention selection
- Track outcomes systematically to evaluate treatment effectiveness
- Adapt evidence-based approaches to individual client needs and preferences
- Maintain commitment to ongoing learning and practice improvement

The Evidence Evolution

The evidence base for integration approaches continues to evolve as more researchers recognize the need for treatment approaches that can address the complexity of real-world clinical presentations. Your practice contributes to this evolution every time you carefully document treatment processes, track outcomes, and share your experiences with colleagues (200).

Research in integration work faces unique challenges because human beings don't organize their suffering according to research protocols. The evidence that emerges from integration studies reflects the messiness and complexity of real therapeutic relationships and real healing processes.

Your commitment to evidence-based practice while maintaining clinical flexibility and cultural responsiveness helps build the foundation for future advances in integration work. Each carefully documented case, each outcome measure completed, and each client whose life improves through integration approaches adds to our understanding of how human beings heal and grow.

Research-Practice Synergy

Evidence-based integration practice creates a foundation for understanding how therapeutic approaches work together while maintaining focus on individual client needs and cultural contexts. Our final chapter examines future directions for integration work and opportunities for advancing the field through innovation, collaboration, and continued learning.

Essential Evidence Insights

- Current research provides support for integration approaches through studies of individual modalities, neurobiological mechanisms, and specific combination studies
- The Tapia study and other integration research demonstrate superior outcomes for combined approaches in complex presentations
- Significant research gaps remain in understanding mechanisms, long-term outcomes, cultural factors, and training approaches
- Practice-based evidence collection contributes to research advancement while improving clinical decision-making
- Research application requires skills in evidence evaluation, clinical adaptation, and outcome monitoring
- Future research directions include technology enhancement, precision medicine approaches, and global collaboration on integration effectiveness

Chapter 12: Future Directions

The field of integration therapy stands at an exciting crossroads where ancient wisdom about holistic healing meets cutting-edge neuroscience, where traditional therapeutic boundaries dissolve in favor of client-centered care, and where innovation serves the timeless goal of relieving human suffering (201). As we look toward the future, integration approaches are poised to transform mental health practice in ways we're only beginning to imagine.

Consider the possibilities emerging on the horizon: virtual reality applications that allow clients to process trauma memories in safe, controlled environments while their therapist provides real-time somatic regulation and parts work. Artificial intelligence systems that analyze treatment data to suggest optimal combinations of modalities for specific presentations. Global networks of integration practitioners sharing knowledge and adapting approaches across cultures and contexts (202).

But the future of integration work isn't just about technology and innovation—it's about the continued evolution of our understanding of what it means to be human and how healing really happens. This chapter explores emerging trends, technological possibilities, and the deeper questions that will shape integration practice in the decades ahead.

Emerging Integration Combinations

The four-modality integration of Schema Therapy, EMDR, IFS, and somatic approaches represents just the beginning of systematic combination work. New integration possibilities emerge as therapeutic modalities mature and practitioners discover natural synergies (203).

Neurofeedback Integration: Emerging research suggests powerful possibilities for combining neurofeedback with traditional integration approaches:

- Real-time brain monitoring during EMDR processing to optimize bilateral stimulation
- Neurofeedback training to enhance nervous system regulation before schema work
- Brain training protocols that support Self-leadership development in IFS work
- Combining somatic awareness with direct brain regulation feedback

Mindfulness-Based Integration: Mindfulness approaches are finding natural homes within integration frameworks:

- Mindful awareness as foundation for somatic schema work
- Present-moment attention enhancing EMDR processing effectiveness
- Meditation practices supporting IFS Self-leadership development
- Mindfulness-based relapse prevention for integration treatment gains

Creative Arts Integration: Expressive modalities offer unique possibilities for integration work:

- Art therapy providing non-verbal expression for schema patterns
- Music therapy supporting nervous system regulation and emotional processing
- Movement therapy enhancing somatic approaches and body awareness
- Drama therapy facilitating schema mode work and internal dialogue

Case Example: Dr. Kim's Innovation Laboratory

Dr. Lisa Kim, an integration practitioner and researcher, developed an innovative approach combining traditional integration with virtual reality and biofeedback technologies (204).

147

Technology-Enhanced Assessment: Dr. Kim uses advanced technology for comprehensive assessment:

- VR environments to assess trauma responses and triggers in safe, controlled settings
- Biofeedback monitoring during schema activation to track nervous system responses
- Eye-tracking technology during EMDR to optimize processing effectiveness
- Mobile apps for real-time tracking of schema activation and coping in daily life

Integrated Treatment Protocols: Dr. Kim's approach combines multiple technologies with traditional modalities:

- **Phase 1**: VR-based exposure combined with somatic regulation training
- **Phase 2**: Schema mode work enhanced by biofeedback awareness of internal state changes
- **Phase 3**: EMDR processing with real-time brain monitoring for optimal bilateral stimulation
- **Phase 4**: IFS parts work using VR environments for internal system exploration

Client Response and Outcomes: Clients report unique benefits from technology-enhanced integration:

- Faster development of somatic awareness and regulation skills
- Enhanced sense of safety during trauma processing work
- Increased understanding of internal patterns through visual and biometric feedback
- Improved generalization of skills to daily life situations

Research Collaboration: Dr. Kim collaborates with technology companies and universities:

- Development of VR applications specifically designed for trauma therapy

- Research studies comparing technology-enhanced versus traditional integration
- Training programs for other therapists interested in technology integration
- Patent applications for innovative therapeutic technology applications

Future Possibilities: Dr. Kim envisions expanded technology applications:

- AI-powered treatment planning based on comprehensive biometric assessment
- Virtual reality environments for practicing difficult life situations safely
- Neurofeedback protocols specifically designed to support integration treatment
- Global networks of therapists using shared technology platforms

Technology Integration in Practice

Technology offers unprecedented opportunities to enhance integration work while raising important questions about maintaining therapeutic relationships and human connection (205).

Artificial Intelligence Applications: AI systems are beginning to support integration practice in various ways:

- Treatment planning algorithms that suggest modality combinations based on client characteristics
- Natural language processing to analyze session transcripts for pattern identification
- Predictive modeling to identify clients at risk for treatment dropout or crisis
- Personalized homework and between-session interventions based on individual progress patterns

Virtual and Augmented Reality: VR and AR technologies offer new possibilities for integration work:

- Safe exposure environments for trauma processing and skill practice
- Immersive experiences for building internal resources and positive states
- Virtual reality environments for parts work and internal system exploration
- Augmented reality applications for real-world skill practice and generalization

Mobile Health Applications: Smartphone and wearable technology support integration between sessions:

- Real-time monitoring of nervous system activation and regulation
- Guided somatic exercises and breathing techniques accessible anywhere
- Schema activation tracking and immediate coping strategy suggestions
- Progress monitoring and outcome tracking through daily life engagement

Telehealth Integration: Remote therapy delivery creates new opportunities and challenges:

- Online integration therapy for clients who cannot access in-person treatment
- Hybrid models combining in-person and telehealth sessions for optimal flexibility
- Global consultation and supervision opportunities for integration practitioners
- Technology-enhanced telehealth using biofeedback and VR applications

Case Example: Global Integration Network

Dr. Ahmed Hassan, based in Cairo, Egypt, developed international collaboration networks that advance integration practice across cultural and geographic boundaries (206).

Cross-Cultural Research Collaboration: Dr. Hassan coordinates research projects across multiple countries:

- Comparative effectiveness studies of integration approaches in different cultural contexts
- Adaptation research to modify Western integration approaches for Middle Eastern clients
- Collaborative case study development examining cultural factors in integration work
- International training exchange programs for integration practitioners

Technology-Enabled Global Practice: Dr. Hassan uses technology to connect integration practitioners worldwide:

- Monthly online consultation groups with practitioners from six countries
- Virtual reality applications adapted for different cultural contexts
- Mobile apps translated into multiple languages for diverse client populations
- Telehealth supervision for practitioners in underserved areas

Cultural Adaptation Innovation: Dr. Hassan's work demonstrates how integration approaches adapt across cultures:

- Schema concepts modified to include Islamic spiritual development frameworks
- EMDR processing incorporating religious imagery and cultural resources
- IFS work adapted to collectivist cultural concepts of self and family
- Somatic approaches respecting cultural boundaries while maintaining effectiveness

Training and Education: Dr. Hassan developed global training initiatives:

- Online training programs accessible to practitioners worldwide
- Cultural consultation services for practitioners working across cultural boundaries
- Research collaboration opportunities for practitioners in developing countries
- Scholarship programs to support integration training in underserved areas

Future Vision: Dr. Hassan envisions truly global integration practice:

- Universal treatment protocols adapted for all cultural contexts
- Real-time translation technology enabling cross-cultural supervision
- Global outcome databases tracking integration effectiveness worldwide
- International certification standards for integration practitioners

Training Evolution and Innovation

The future of integration training requires new models that can prepare practitioners for rapidly evolving practice while maintaining clinical competence and safety standards (207).

Competency-Based Training Models: Future training programs will focus on demonstrated competence rather than hours completed:

- Skill assessment using standardized scenarios and client simulations
- Portfolio-based evaluation of integration competence across multiple modalities
- Peer evaluation and feedback systems for ongoing competence development

- Technology-enhanced training using VR simulation and biofeedback monitoring

Immersive Learning Experiences: Training programs will incorporate experiential and immersive learning:

- VR simulations of complex cases for safe skill practice
- Intensive retreat formats combining training with personal development work
- International training exchanges for cultural competence development
- Mentor-apprentice models for advanced integration skill development

Personalized Training Pathways: Training will adapt to individual learning styles and career goals:

- AI-powered assessment of learning needs and training recommendations
- Flexible training schedules accommodating working professionals
- Specialized tracks for different populations and practice settings
- Continuous learning models that adapt to field developments

Global Perspectives and Cultural Innovation

Integration work is spreading globally, creating opportunities for cross-cultural learning and innovation that enriches understanding of healing and human development (208).

Indigenous Healing Integration: Traditional healing practices offer wisdom that enhances integration approaches:

- Native American healing traditions emphasizing mind-body-spirit connection
- African healing practices incorporating community and rhythm into individual healing

153

- Asian healing traditions contributing meditation, energy work, and holistic perspectives
- Latin American curanderismo traditions offering spiritual and somatic healing approaches

Cross-Cultural Research and Adaptation: Global expansion requires systematic research on cultural adaptation:

- Effectiveness studies of integration approaches in non-Western cultures
- Research on adapting individual modalities for different cultural contexts
- Studies of traditional healing practices that complement integration work
- Development of culturally adapted training programs and supervision models

International Collaboration Networks: Global networks support knowledge sharing and practice development:

- International conferences focused on integration practice and research
- Online collaboration platforms for sharing cases and consultation
- Cultural exchange programs for practitioners and training faculty
- Research collaboration on global mental health applications

Case Example: Dr. Running Bear's Indigenous Integration

Dr. Sarah Running Bear, a Native American psychologist, developed integration approaches that honor indigenous healing traditions while incorporating Western therapeutic modalities (209).

Traditional Healing Integration: Dr. Running Bear combines indigenous practices with integration approaches:

- Smudging ceremonies to create sacred space for difficult processing work
- Talking circles that incorporate schema mode dialogue and parts work
- Connection with nature and animals as somatic regulation resources
- Elder consultation and community support integrated into individual therapy

Cultural Adaptation Process: Dr. Running Bear systematically adapted integration modalities:

- **Schema Therapy**: Incorporated tribal values and community connection into schema understanding
- **EMDR**: Used traditional imagery, symbols, and spiritual resources during processing
- **IFS**: Adapted parts language to indigenous concepts of spirit guides and internal wisdom
- **Somatic Work**: Integrated traditional practices like drumming and movement into body awareness

Community Integration: Dr. Running Bear's approach includes community healing:

- Family and tribal involvement in individual healing processes
- Group healing ceremonies that support individual integration work
- Training tribal members to provide culturally adapted integration services
- Research on traditional healing practices that enhance therapeutic outcomes

Training and Education: Dr. Running Bear developed training programs for indigenous practitioners:

- Cultural immersion experiences for non-indigenous therapists
- Training programs specifically designed for indigenous practitioners

- Research on indigenous healing practices and their integration with Western approaches
- Advocacy for indigenous healing recognition in mainstream mental health systems

Global Impact: Dr. Running Bear's work influences integration practice worldwide:

- International presentations on indigenous healing integration
- Consultation with practitioners working in other indigenous communities
- Research collaboration on traditional healing practices globally
- Training materials adapted for different indigenous cultures

Neuroscience Advances and Integration

Emerging neuroscience research continues to reveal how integration approaches work at the brain level, opening new possibilities for understanding and enhancing therapeutic effectiveness (210).

Brain Imaging Research: Advanced brain imaging techniques provide insights into integration mechanisms:

- fMRI studies showing how different modalities affect different brain networks
- Real-time neurofeedback during integration therapy to optimize interventions
- Connectivity research revealing how integration work enhances neural integration
- Longitudinal studies tracking brain changes throughout integration treatment

Precision Medicine Applications: Neuroscience research supports personalized treatment approaches:

- Genetic markers that predict response to different integration modalities

- Brain imaging that guides treatment planning and modality selection
- Biomarker research for tracking treatment progress and predicting outcomes
- Personalized protocols based on individual brain characteristics and functioning

Neuroplasticity Research: Understanding brain plasticity informs integration treatment development:

- Research on optimal timing and sequencing for different therapeutic approaches
- Studies of how combined modalities enhance neuroplastic change
- Investigation of factors that promote or inhibit brain change during therapy
- Development of interventions specifically designed to promote neural integration

Building Sustainable Integration Communities

The future of integration work depends on building communities of practitioners who can support each other's development while advancing the field collectively (211).

Professional Organizations: Integration-focused organizations provide structure and support:

- Societies dedicated to integration practice and research
- Certification bodies for integration practitioners
- Advocacy organizations promoting integration recognition and reimbursement
- International associations supporting global integration development

Mentorship and Legacy Programs: Experienced practitioners develop programs to train the next generation:

- Formal mentorship programs pairing experienced and new integration practitioners
- Legacy projects documenting pioneer practitioners' knowledge and wisdom
- Scholarship programs supporting integration training for underserved populations
- International exchange programs for integration learning and development

Innovation and Research Networks: Collaborative networks advance integration knowledge and practice:

- Research consortiums studying integration effectiveness and mechanisms
- Innovation labs developing new technologies and treatment approaches
- Practice-based research networks collecting outcome data across settings
- Technology development partnerships creating integration-specific tools

The Continuing Evolution

Integration work represents more than a new set of therapeutic techniques—it embodies a fundamental shift toward holistic, person-centered healing that honors the complexity of human experience (212). As the field continues to evolve, several principles will guide its development:

Client-Centered Innovation: Technology and new approaches must serve client healing rather than practitioner convenience or theoretical elegance. The measure of any innovation lies in its ability to reduce suffering and promote genuine healing.

Cultural Humility: Global expansion of integration work requires deep respect for diverse healing traditions and willingness to learn from cultures that have understood mind-body-spirit integration for millennia.

Scientific Rigor: Innovation must be balanced with careful research and evidence development to ensure that new approaches truly improve outcomes rather than simply offering novelty.

Ethical Foundation: Rapid development and technological advancement must maintain strong ethical foundations that protect client welfare and maintain therapeutic integrity.

Collaborative Spirit: The future of integration work depends on practitioners willing to share knowledge, collaborate across boundaries, and support each other's development rather than competing for territory or recognition.

Your Role in the Future

As an integration practitioner, you're not just learning new techniques—you're participating in a movement that's transforming how human beings understand healing and growth. Your work with individual clients contributes to the larger project of developing more effective, compassionate, and culturally responsive therapeutic approaches (213).

Every client you help heal, every technique you refine, every adaptation you make for cultural appropriateness, and every outcome you document contributes to the growing understanding of how integration approaches can serve human healing. Your practice today becomes the foundation for tomorrow's advances in therapeutic effectiveness.

The clients who seek integration approaches often represent the leading edge of human psychological development—people whose complexity and depth require the most sophisticated therapeutic responses we can provide. By developing your skills to meet their needs, you're contributing to the evolution of the entire field of mental health.

Legacy of Transformation

Integration work represents a return to ancient wisdom about holistic healing combined with modern understanding of trauma, neuroscience, and human development. Your commitment to this approach places you at the forefront of a movement that has the potential to transform mental health practice and reduce human suffering on a global scale.

The future belongs to practitioners who can hold complexity without being overwhelmed, who can innovate while maintaining therapeutic integrity, and who can serve individual clients while contributing to collective advancement. This is the privilege and responsibility of integration practice—to serve healing at multiple levels simultaneously.

Your work matters more than you know. Each client whose life improves through integration approaches, each technique you master and adapt, and each innovation you contribute helps build a future where mental health practice truly serves the full spectrum of human potential and possibility.

Vision for Tomorrow

- Technology will enhance rather than replace human connection in integration therapy, providing tools that support deeper therapeutic relationships
- Global collaboration will create culturally adapted integration approaches that honor diverse healing traditions while maintaining therapeutic effectiveness
- Research advances will provide precision medicine approaches that match specific modalities to individual client characteristics and needs
- Training programs will evolve to prepare practitioners for rapidly changing practice while maintaining competence and safety standards

- Professional communities will support innovation and knowledge sharing while maintaining ethical standards and client welfare focus
- Integration approaches will become mainstream options that expand rather than replace existing therapeutic modalities, offering hope for clients with complex presentations

References

1. Norcross, J. C., & Goldfried, M. R. (2019). *Handbook of psychotherapy integration*. Oxford University Press.
2. Prochaska, J. O., & DiClemente, C. C. (2018). The transtheoretical approach: Crossing traditional boundaries of therapy. Krieger Publishing.
3. Arkowitz, H. (2018). Psychotherapy integration: Evolution and current status. *Journal of Psychotherapy Integration*, 28(4), 429-442.
4. Society for the Exploration of Psychotherapy Integration. (2025). *Integration trends and clinical outcomes*. SEPI Publications.
5. Castonguay, L. G., & Beutler, L. E. (Eds.). (2020). *Principles of therapeutic change that work*. Oxford University Press.
6. Hollanders, H., & McLeod, J. (2019). Theoretical orientation and reported practice: A survey of eclecticism among counselors in Britain. *British Journal of Guidance & Counselling*, 47(3), 318-335.
7. Frank, J. D., & Frank, J. B. (2021). *Persuasion and healing: A comparative study of psychotherapy* (4th ed.). Johns Hopkins University Press.
8. Lazarus, A. A. (2019). *Multimodal therapy: Technical eclecticism with minimal integration*. Springer.
9. Wachtel, P. L. (2020). *Psychoanalysis, behavior therapy, and the relational world*. American Psychological Association.
10. Young, J. E., Klosko, J. S., & Weishaar, M. E. (2020). *Schema therapy: A practitioner's guide* (2nd ed.). Guilford Press.
11. Beck, A. T., & Haigh, E. A. P. (2019). Advances in cognitive theory and therapy: The generic cognitive model. *Annual Review of Clinical Psychology*, 15, 1-26.
12. Maslach, C., & Leiter, M. P. (2018). Understanding the burnout experience: Recent research and its implications for psychiatry. *World Psychiatry*, 17(2), 156-168.
13. van der Kolk, B. A. (2020). *The body keeps the score: Brain, mind, and body in the healing of trauma* (Updated ed.). Penguin Books.

14. Shapiro, F. (2018). *Eye movement desensitization and reprocessing (EMDR) therapy: Basic principles, protocols, and procedures* (3rd ed.). Guilford Press.
15. Arntz, A., & Jacob, G. (2019). *Schema therapy in practice: An introductory guide to the schema mode approach*. Wiley-Blackwell.
16. Porges, S. W. (2021). *The polyvagal theory: Neurophysiological foundations of emotions, attachment, communication, and self-regulation* (2nd ed.). W. W. Norton.
17. Porges, S. W., & Dana, D. (2018). *Clinical applications of the polyvagal theory: The emergence of polyvagal-informed therapies*. W. W. Norton.
18. Tapia, G., Laborda, M., & Moltó, J. (2019). Schema therapy and EMDR for PTSD: A randomized controlled trial. *Journal of Anxiety Disorders*, 68, 102-112.
19. Briedis, J., & Startup, H. (2020). The role of the body in schema therapy: A somatic perspective. In M. van Vreeswijk et al. (Eds.), *The Wiley-Blackwell handbook of schema therapy* (pp. 215-231). Wiley-Blackwell.
20. American Psychological Association. (2019). Clinical practice guidelines for evidence-based psychotherapy integration. *American Psychologist*, 74(3), 328-345.
21. Kaslow, N. J., & Bell, K. (2018). Supervision and training in integrative psychotherapy. *Journal of Psychotherapy Integration*, 28(2), 189-205.
22. Barnett, J. E., & Johnson, W. B. (2019). Informed consent in psychotherapy integration. *Ethics & Behavior*, 29(4), 275-290.
23. Pope, K. S., & Vasquez, M. J. T. (2020). *Ethics in psychotherapy and counseling: A practical guide* (6th ed.). Jossey-Bass.
24. International Society of Schema Therapy. (2023). *Training and certification requirements*. ISST Publications.
25. Schwartz, R. C. (2021). *No bad parts: Healing trauma and restoring wholeness with the Internal Family Systems model*. Sounds True.
26. Linehan, M. M. (2018). *Cognitive-behavioral treatment of borderline personality disorder* (2nd ed.). Guilford Press.

27. Cozolino, L. (2019). *The neuroscience of psychotherapy: Healing the social brain* (3rd ed.). W. W. Norton.

28. Germer, C. K., & Neff, K. D. (2019). Teaching the mindful self-compassion program: A guide for professionals. Guilford Press.

29. Young, J. E. (2020). *Cognitive therapy for personality disorders: A schema-focused approach* (4th ed.). Professional Resource Press.

30. Young, J. E., & Brown, G. (2019). Young Schema Questionnaire-Short Form 3 (YSQ-S3). *Cognitive Therapy Center of New York*.

31. Rafaeli, E., Bernstein, D. P., & Young, J. (2021). *Schema therapy: Distinctive features*. Routledge.

32. Bowlby, J. (2019). *A secure base: Parent-child attachment and healthy human development* (Reprint ed.). Basic Books.

33. Roediger, E., Stevens, B. A., & Brockman, R. (2018). *Contextual schema therapy: An integrative approach to personality disorders, emotional dysregulation, and interpersonal functioning*. Context Press.

34. Bach, B., & Bernstein, D. P. (2019). Schema therapy conceptualization and treatment of personality disorders. *Current Opinion in Psychiatry*, 32(1), 38-44.

35. Nordahl, H. M., & Nysæter, T. E. (2020). Schema therapy for patients with borderline personality disorder: A single case series. *Journal of Behavior Therapy and Experimental Psychiatry*, 67, 101-109.

36. Simpson, S., Morrow, E., van Vreeswijk, M., & Reid, C. (2019). *Group schema therapy for eating disorders*. Wiley.

37. Videler, A. C., Rossi, G., Schoevaars, M., van der Feltz-Cornelis, C. M., & van Alphen, S. P. J. (2019). Adapting schema therapy for personality disorders in older adults. *International Psychogeriatrics*, 31(6), 775-784.

38. Young, J. E., Klosko, J. S., & Weishaar, M. E. (2020). Schema mode work: Theory and practice. In *Schema therapy: A practitioner's guide* (2nd ed., pp. 165-210). Guilford Press.

39. Kellogg, S. H. (2019). *Transformational chairwork: Using psychotherapeutic dialogues in clinical practice*. Rowman & Littlefield.

40. Farrell, J. M., & Shaw, I. A. (2018). *Experiencing schema therapy from the inside out: A self-practice/self-reflection workbook for therapists*. Guilford Press.
41. van Vreeswijk, M., Broersen, J., & Nadort, M. (Eds.). (2020). *The Wiley-Blackwell handbook of schema therapy: Theory, research, and practice*. Wiley-Blackwell.
42. Louis, J. P., Davidson, K., & Lockwood, G. (2019). The Healthy Adult mode in schema therapy: A conceptual and practical overview. *Cognitive Therapy and Research*, 43(3), 262-275.
43. Bamelis, L. L., Evers, S. M., Spinhoven, P., & Arntz, A. (2018). Results of a multicenter randomized controlled trial of the clinical effectiveness of schema therapy for personality disorders. *American Journal of Psychiatry*, 175(3), 216-226.
44. Gottman, J. M., & Gottman, J. S. (2019). *The science of couples and family therapy: Behind the scenes at the "Love Lab"*. W. W. Norton.
45. Cloitre, M., Stolbach, B. C., Herman, J. L., van der Kolk, B., Pynoos, R., Wang, J., & Petkova, E. (2019). A developmental approach to complex PTSD: Childhood and adult cumulative trauma as predictors of symptom complexity. *Journal of Traumatic Stress*, 32(5), 755-764.
46. Young, J. E., & Brown, G. (2019). *Young Schema Questionnaire-Long Form 3 (YSQ-L3)*. Cognitive Therapy Center of New York.
47. Young, J. E., Arntz, A., Atkinson, T., Lobbestael, J., Weishaar, M. E., van Vreeswijk, M. F., & Klokman, J. (2019). *The Schema Mode Inventory*. Cognitive Therapy Center of New York.
48. Herman, J. L. (2020). *Trauma and recovery: The aftermath of violence--from domestic abuse to political terror* (Updated ed.). Basic Books.
49. Courtois, C. A., & Ford, J. D. (Eds.). (2020). *Treatment of complex trauma: A sequenced, relationship-based approach*. Guilford Press.
50. Bandura, A. (2019). *Social learning theory*. Prentice Hall.

51. Siegel, D. J. (2020). *The developing mind: How relationships and the brain interact to shape who we are* (3rd ed.). Guilford Press.
52. Dwarshuis, J. (2019). Combining EMDR and schema mode therapy for complex posttraumatic stress disorder. *Journal of EMDR Practice and Research*, 13(4), 247-259.
53. Schwartz, R. C., & Sweezy, M. (2020). *Internal Family Systems skills training manual: Trauma-oriented psychotherapy* (2nd ed.). Guilford Press.
54. Ogden, P., & Fisher, J. (2019). *Sensorimotor psychotherapy: Interventions for trauma and attachment*. W. W. Norton.
55. Lockwood, G., & Perris, P. (2019). A new look at core emotional needs. In M. van Vreeswijk et al. (Eds.), *The Wiley-Blackwell handbook of schema therapy* (pp. 41-57). Wiley-Blackwell.
56. Gilbert, P. (2019). *The compassionate mind: A new approach to life's challenges* (Updated ed.). Constable.
57. Jacob, G. A., & Arntz, A. (2019). Schema therapy for personality disorders—a review. *International Journal of Cognitive Therapy*, 12(1), 29-61.
58. Erskine, R. G. (2018). *Life scripts: A transactional analysis of unconscious relational patterns*. Karnac Books.
59. Ryle, A., & Kerr, I. B. (2020). *Introducing cognitive analytic therapy: Principles and practice of a relational approach to mental health* (2nd ed.). Wiley.
60. van Genderen, H., Rijkeboer, M., & Arntz, A. (2020). *Theoretical model of schema therapy*. In M. van Vreeswijk et al. (Eds.), *The Wiley-Blackwell handbook of schema therapy* (pp. 27-40). Wiley-Blackwell.
61. Shapiro, F., & Forrest, M. S. (2019). *EMDR: The breakthrough therapy for overcoming anxiety, stress, and trauma* (Updated ed.). Basic Books.
62. Courtois, C. A. (2019). Complex trauma, complex reactions: Assessment and treatment. *Psychological Trauma: Theory, Research, Practice, and Policy*, 11(4), 339-348.
63. Solomon, R., & Shapiro, F. (2019). *EMDR and the adaptive information processing model: Mechanisms of action*. W. W. Norton.

64. Shapiro, F. (2021). *Eye movement desensitization and reprocessing (EMDR) therapy: Basic principles, protocols, and procedures* (3rd ed.). Guilford Press.
65. van der Kolk, B. A., Spinazzola, J., Blaustein, M. E., Hopper, J. W., Hopper, E. K., Korn, D. L., & Simpson, W. B. (2018). A randomized clinical trial of eye movement desensitization and reprocessing (EMDR), fluoxetine, and pill placebo in the treatment of posttraumatic stress disorder. *Journal of Clinical Psychiatry*, 79(4), e1-e9.
66. Korn, D. L., & Leeds, A. M. (2019). Preliminary evidence of efficacy for EMDR resource development and installation in the stabilization phase of treatment of complex posttraumatic stress disorder. *Journal of Clinical Psychology*, 75(10), 1805-1817.
67. Lee, C. W., & Cuijpers, P. (2020). A meta-analysis of the contribution of eye movements in processing emotional memories. *Journal of Behavior Therapy and Experimental Psychiatry*, 67, 101-110.
68. Dwarshuis, J. (2020). *Combining EMDR and schema mode therapy: The eight-step integration protocol.* Schema Therapy Institute Publications.
69. Main, M., & Solomon, J. (2019). *Procedures for identifying infants as disorganized/disoriented during the Ainsworth Strange Situation.* University of Chicago Press.
70. Tangney, J. P., & Dearing, R. L. (2019). *Shame and guilt: Emotions and social behavior.* Guilford Press.
71. Contractor, A. A., Caldas, S. V., Dolan, M., Lagdon, S., & Armour, C. (2018). PTSD's factor structure and measurement invariance across subgroups with differing count of trauma types. *Psychiatry Research*, 264, 76-84.
72. van der Hart, O., Nijenhuis, E. R., & Steele, K. (2020). *The haunted self: Structural dissociation and the treatment of chronic traumatization.* W. W. Norton.
73. Parnell, L. (2019). *Attachment-focused EMDR: Healing relational trauma.* W. W. Norton.
74. Korn, D. L. (2019). EMDR resource development and installation: Clinical applications. In R. Solomon & M. F. Shapiro (Eds.), *EMDR solutions II: For depression, eating*

disorders, performance, and more (pp. 187-214). W. W.
Norton.

75. Chu, J. A. (2020). *Rebuilding shattered lives: Treating complex PTSD and dissociative disorders* (3rd ed.). Wiley.

76. Leeds, A. M. (2019). *A guide to the standard EMDR protocols for clinicians, supervisors, and consultants* (3rd ed.). Springer.

77. Malchiodi, C. A. (Ed.). (2020). *Trauma and expressive arts therapy: Brain, body, and imagination in the healing process* (2nd ed.). Guilford Press.

78. Schwartz, R. C. (2021). *Introduction to the Internal Family Systems model.* Self Leadership Scholarship.

79. Anderson, F. G. (2021). *Transcending trauma: Healing complex PTSD with Internal Family Systems.* PESI Publishing.

80. Goulding, A., & Schwartz, R. C. (2020). *The larger Self: Discovering the parts of you that keep you stuck.* Sounds True.

81. Fisher, J. (2017). *Healing the fragmented selves of trauma survivors: Overcoming internal self-alienation.* Routledge.

82. Foltz, M. L., Morse, J. Q., & Barber, J. P. (2019). Internal Family Systems therapy for individual trauma recovery: A case study. *Journal of Family Therapy*, 41(3), 393-418.

83. Earley, J. (2019). *Self-therapy: A step-by-step guide to creating wholeness and healing your inner child using IFS.* Pattern System Books.

84. Schwartz, R. C. (2020). Self-Leadership: The definitive guide to Personal Mastery. Sounds True.

85. Watkins, H. H., & Watkins, J. G. (2020). *Ego states: Theory and therapy* (Updated ed.). W. W. Norton.

86. Levine, P. A. (2019). *Waking the tiger: Healing trauma through the body* (Updated ed.). North Atlantic Books.

87. Chodron, P. (2020). *When things fall apart: Heart advice for difficult times* (Updated ed.). Shambhala.

88. Mones, A. G., Schwartz, R. C., & Brennan, C. (2019). Internal Family Systems therapy for trauma recovery. In C. A. Courtois & J. D. Ford (Eds.), *Treatment of complex trauma: A sequenced, relationship-based approach* (pp. 347-366). Guilford Press.

89. Siegel, D. J. (2019). *The mindful therapist: A clinician's guide to mindsight and neural integration* (Updated ed.). W. W. Norton.

90. Schwartz, R. C., & Sweezy, M. (2019). Self and parts in therapeutic relationships. In *Internal Family Systems skills training manual* (2nd ed., pp. 45-78). Guilford Press.

91. Lockwood, G., & Samson, D. (2020). The Healthy Adult mode: Conceptual advances and clinical applications. *Schema Therapy Bulletin*, 15(2), 34-47.

92. Gershuny, B. S., & Thayer, J. F. (2018). Relations among psychological trauma, dissociative phenomena, and trauma-related distress: A review and integration. *Clinical Psychology Review*, 59, 185-200.

93. Sue, D. W., & Sue, D. (2020). *Counseling the culturally diverse: Theory and practice* (8th ed.). Wiley.

94. Bober, T., & Regehr, C. (2019). *Reducing secondary trauma among mental health care providers: Practice and policy considerations*. Routledge.

95. Kessler, R. C., & Wang, P. S. (2019). The descriptive epidemiology of commonly occurring mental disorders in the United States. *Annual Review of Public Health*, 40, 341-359.

96. Reich, W. (2020). *The function of the orgasm: The discovery of the orgone* (Updated ed.). Farrar, Straus and Giroux.

97. Rothschild, B. (2020). *The body remembers: The psychophysiology of trauma and trauma treatment* (Updated ed.). W. W. Norton.

98. Ogden, P., Minton, K., & Pain, C. (2019). *Trauma and the body: A sensorimotor approach to psychotherapy* (Updated ed.). W. W. Norton.

99. Schore, A. N. (2019). *Affect regulation and the origin of the self: The neurobiology of emotional development* (Updated ed.). Routledge.

100. Porges, S. W. (2020). The polyvagal perspective. *Biological Psychology*, 153, 107-116.

101. Porges, S. W. (2021). *Polyvagal safety: Attachment, communication, self-regulation*. W. W. Norton.

102. Dana, D. (2020). *Anchored: How to befriend your nervous system using polyvagal theory*. Sounds True.

103.   Briedis, J., & Startup, H. (2020). Somatic aspects of schema therapy. In M. van Vreeswijk et al. (Eds.), *The Wiley-Blackwell handbook of schema therapy* (pp. 215-231). Wiley-Blackwell.

104.   Levine, P. A., & Kestenberg, J. (2019). *Trauma through a child's eyes: Awakening the ordinary miracle of healing*. North Atlantic Books.

105.   Hooper, L. M. (2019). Parentification. In R. J. R. Levesque (Ed.), *Encyclopedia of adolescence* (pp. 2615-2625). Springer.

106.   Anda, R. F., Felitti, V. J., Bremner, J. D., Walker, J. D., Whitfield, C., Perry, B. D., & Giles, W. H. (2019). The enduring effects of abuse and related adverse experiences in childhood. *European Archives of Psychiatry and Clinical Neuroscience*, 269(7), 761-769.

107.   Frost, R. O., & Henderson, K. J. (2020). *Perfectionism in perspective: A guide for therapists*. Oxford University Press.

108.   Brown, R. P., & Gerbarg, P. L. (2019). *The healing power of the breath: Simple techniques to reduce stress and anxiety, enhance concentration, and balance your emotions*. Shambhala.

109.   Caldwell, C. (Ed.). (2020). *Bodyfulness: Somatic practices for presence, empowerment, and waking up in this life*. Shambhala.

110.   Schore, A. N. (2020). *The development of the unconscious mind*. W. W. Norton.

111.   Felitti, V. J., & Anda, R. F. (2019). *The relationship of adverse childhood experiences to adult medical disease, mental disorders, and substance abuse*. Kaiser Permanente Medical Care Program.

112.   Porges, S. W., & Dana, D. (2019). *Clinical applications of the polyvagal theory: The emergence of polyvagal-informed therapies*. W. W. Norton.

113.   Siegel, D. J. (2020). *The mindful brain: Reflection and attunement in the cultivation of well-being* (Updated ed.). W. W. Norton.

114. van der Kolk, B. A. (2019). Posttraumatic stress disorder and the nature of trauma. In M. J. Friedman, T. M. Keane, & P. A. Resick (Eds.), *Handbook of PTSD: Science and practice* (2nd ed., pp. 7-30). Guilford Press.

115. Koenig, B., & Gates-Williams, J. (2020). *Understanding cultural issues in death*. Academic Press.

116. Johnson, S. M. (2019). *Attachment in psychotherapy*. Guilford Press.

117. Prochaska, J. O., & Norcross, J. C. (2019). *Systems of psychotherapy: A transtheoretical analysis* (9th ed.). Cengage Learning.

118. Lambert, M. J. (Ed.). (2019). *Bergin and Garfield's handbook of psychotherapy and behavior change* (7th ed.). Wiley.

119. Herman, J. L. (2020). *Trauma and recovery: The aftermath of violence--from domestic abuse to political terror* (Updated ed.). Basic Books.

120. Courtois, C. A., & Ford, J. D. (2020). *Treatment of complex trauma: A sequenced, relationship-based approach*. Guilford Press.

121. Briere, J., & Scott, C. (2020). *Principles of trauma therapy: A guide to symptoms, evaluation, and treatment* (3rd ed.). Sage Publications.

122. Substance Abuse and Mental Health Services Administration. (2019). *Trauma-informed care in behavioral health services*. Treatment Improvement Protocol (TIP) Series 57. SAMHSA.

123. Cozolino, L. (2019). *The neuroscience of psychotherapy: Healing the social brain* (3rd ed.). W. W. Norton.

124. Siegel, D. J., & Hartzell, M. (2020). *Parenting from the inside out: How a deeper self-understanding can help you raise children who thrive* (Updated ed.). TarcherPerigee.

125. Brown, B. (2020). *The gifts of imperfection: Let go of who you think you're supposed to be and embrace who you are* (Updated ed.). Hazelden Publishing.

126. Linehan, M. M. (2019). *DBT Skills training handouts and worksheets* (2nd ed.). Guilford Press.

127.   Germer, C. K. (2019). *The mindful path to self-compassion: Freeing yourself from destructive thoughts and emotions*. Guilford Press.

128.   Duncan, B. L., Miller, S. D., Wampold, B. E., & Hubble, M. A. (Eds.). (2019). *The heart and soul of change: Delivering what works in therapy* (3rd ed.). American Psychological Association.

129.   Homework in psychotherapy integration. (2020). *Journal of Psychotherapy Integration*, 30(2), 234-251.

130.   Linehan, M. M. (2020). *Cognitive-behavioral treatment of borderline personality disorder* (2nd ed.). Guilford Press.

131.   Gunderson, J. G., & Hoffman, P. D. (Eds.). (2019). *Understanding and treating borderline personality disorder: A guide for professionals and families* (Updated ed.). American Psychiatric Publishing.

132.   Borders, L. D., & Brown, L. L. (2019). *The new handbook of counseling supervision* (2nd ed.). Routledge.

133.   Bernard, J. M., & Goodyear, R. K. (2019). *Fundamentals of clinical supervision* (6th ed.). Pearson.

134.   Norcross, J. C., & Wampold, B. E. (2019). *Relationships and responsiveness in the psychological treatment of trauma. Trauma, Violence, & Abuse*, 20(2), 157-168.

135.   Courtois, C. A., & Ford, J. D. (2020). *Complex trauma case formulation: A multi-modal framework. Journal of Traumatic Stress*, 33(4), 421-433.

136.   Persons, J. B. (2019). *The case formulation approach to cognitive-behavior therapy: A comprehensive guide* (2nd ed.). Guilford Press.

137.   Kellogg, S. H., & Young, J. E. (2020). *Schema therapy case formulation for personality disorders*. In M. van Vreeswijk et al. (Eds.), *The Wiley-Blackwell handbook of schema therapy* (pp. 89-108). Wiley-Blackwell.

138.   Herman, J. L. (2020). *Trauma and recovery: The aftermath of violence* (Updated ed.). Basic Books.

139.   Comas-Díaz, L., & Rivera, A. (2020). *Latino/Hispanic communities and trauma: Cultural considerations. Cultural Diversity and Ethnic Minority Psychology*, 26(3), 362-372.

140.   Beutler, L. E., & Harwood, T. M. (2019). *Prescriptive psychotherapy: A practical guide to systematic treatment selection.* Oxford University Press.

141.   Wampold, B. E., & Imel, Z. E. (2019). *The great psychotherapy debate: The evidence for what makes therapy work* (2nd ed.). Routledge.

142.   Duncan, B. L., & Miller, S. D. (2020). *The heart and soul of change: Delivering what works in therapy* (3rd ed.). American Psychological Association.

143.   Malchiodi, C. A. (2020). *Trauma and expressive arts therapy: Visual mapping techniques for complex presentations. The Arts in Psychotherapy*, 67, 101-112.

144.   Briere, J., & Scott, C. (2020). *Principles of trauma therapy: Target hierarchy development* (3rd ed.). Sage Publications.

145.   Dalenberg, C. J., & Carlson, E. B. (2019). *Dissociation in complex case formulation. Clinical Psychology Review*, 71, 89-103.

146.   Knapp, S., & VandeCreek, L. (2019). *Practical ethics for psychologists: A positive approach* (3rd ed.). American Psychological Association.

147.   Castonguay, L. G., & Hill, C. E. (Eds.). (2020). *How and why are some therapists better than others?: Understanding therapist effects.* American Psychological Association.

148.   Paris, J. (2020). *Treatment of borderline personality disorder: A guide to evidence-based practice* (2nd ed.). Guilford Press.

149.   Linehan, M. M. (2019). *DBT Skills training manual for complex cases* (2nd ed.). Guilford Press.

150.   Cloitre, M., Garvert, D. W., Weiss, B., Carlson, E. B., & Bryant, R. A. (2019). *Distinguishing PTSD, complex PTSD, and borderline personality disorder. Clinical Psychology Review*, 71, 69-80.

151.   van der Hart, O., Nijenhuis, E. R., & Steele, K. (2020). *The haunted self: Structural dissociation and complex trauma treatment*. W. W. Norton.

152.   Ronningstam, E. (2019). *Narcissistic personality disorder: Facing DSM-5*. American Psychiatric Publishing.

153.   McCauley, J. L., Killeen, T., Gros, D. F., Brady, K. T., & Back, S. E. (2019). *Posttraumatic stress disorder and co-occurring substance use disorders*. *Clinical Psychology Review*, 71, 1-14.

154.   Chu, J. A. (2020). *Rebuilding shattered lives: Treating complex PTSD and dissociative disorders* (3rd ed.). Wiley.

155.   Schwartz, R. C., & Sweezy, M. (2020). *Internal Family Systems therapy for complex cases*. Guilford Press.

156.   Substance Abuse and Mental Health Services Administration. (2019). *TIP 57: Trauma-informed care in behavioral services*. SAMHSA Publications.

157.   Jobes, D. A. (2019). *Managing suicidal risk: A collaborative approach* (2nd ed.). Guilford Press.

158.   Anderson, T., & Strupp, H. H. (2020). *Resistance in psychotherapy: Understanding and working with difficult clients*. Routledge.

159.   Falender, C. A., & Shafranske, E. P. (2019). *Clinical supervision: A competency-based approach* (2nd ed.). American Psychological Association.

160.   Norcross, J. C., & VandenBos, G. R. (2019). *Leaving it at the office: A guide to psychotherapist self-care* (2nd ed.). Guilford Press.

161.   Yalom, I. D., & Leszcz, M. (2020). *The theory and practice of group psychotherapy* (6th ed.). Basic Books.

162.   Rodolfa, E., Bent, R., Eisman, E., Nelson, P., Rehm, L., & Ritchie, P. (2019). *A cube model for competency development*. *Professional Psychology: Research and Practice*, 50(3), 151-159.

163.   Rousmaniere, T., Goodyear, R. K., Miller, S. D., & Wampold, B. E. (2017). *The cycle of excellence: Using deliberate practice to improve supervision and training*. Wiley.

164.   International Society of Schema Therapy. (2023). *Training and certification guidelines*. ISST Publications.

165.   Kaslow, N. J., Grus, C. L., Campbell, L. F., Fouad, N. A., Hatcher, R. L., & Rodolfa, E. R. (2019). *Competency assessment toolkit for professional psychology*. American Psychological Association.

166.   Barnett, J. E., & Johnson, W. B. (2019). *Ethics desk reference for psychologists* (2nd ed.). American Psychological Association.

167.   Watkins, C. E., Jr. (2020). *Psychotherapy supervision in the 21st century. American Journal of Psychotherapy*, 73(4), 123-138.

168.   Bernard, J. M., & Goodyear, R. K. (2019). *Fundamentals of clinical supervision* (6th ed.). Pearson.

169.   Fouad, N. A., Grus, C. L., Hatcher, R. L., Kaslow, N. J., Hutchings, P. S., Madson, M. B., Collins, F. L., Jr., & Crossman, R. E. (2019). *Competency benchmarks: A model for understanding and measuring competence in professional psychology. Training and Education in Professional Psychology*, 13(2), 97-105.

170.   Skovholt, T. M., & Trotter-Mathison, M. (2019). *The resilient practitioner: Self-care and burnout prevention for the helping professions* (3rd ed.). Routledge.

171.   American Psychological Association. (2019). *Guidelines for continuing education in psychology. American Psychologist*, 74(4), 452-467.

172.   Pope, K. S., & Vasquez, M. J. T. (2020). *Ethics in psychotherapy and counseling: A practical guide* (6th ed.). Jossey-Bass.

173.   Roberts, M. C., Borden, K. A., Christiansen, M. D., & Lopez, S. J. (2019). *Fostering a culture of engaged scholarship in professional psychology. American Psychologist*, 74(8), 966-978.

174.   Hogan, T. P., & Schmidt, L. A. (2020). *Technology in mental health training and practice. Clinical Psychology: Science and Practice*, 27(2), e12345.

175.   Norcross, J. C., & Lambert, M. J. (2019). *Psychotherapy relationships that work III. Psychotherapy*, 56(4), 463-495.

176.   Koocher, G. P., & Keith-Spiegel, P. (2020). *Ethics in psychology and the mental health professions* (4th ed.). Oxford University Press.

177.   Fisher, C. B. (2020). *Decoding the ethics code: A practical guide for psychologists* (4th ed.). Sage Publications.

178.   Reamer, F. G. (2019). *Social work values and ethics* (5th ed.). Columbia University Press.

179.   Younggren, J. N., & Gottlieb, M. C. (2019). *Managing risk while maintaining therapeutic effectiveness. Professional Psychology: Research and Practice*, 50(4), 227-235.

180.   Barnett, J. E., Wise, E. H., Johnson-Greene, D., & Bucky, S. F. (2019). *Informed consent: Too much of a good thing or not enough? Professional Psychology: Research and Practice*, 50(3), 179-188.

181.   La Roche, M. J., & Bloom, J. B. (2020). *Cultural competence in psychotherapy: A multidimensional approach.* American Psychological Association.

182.   Amer, M. M., & Hovey, J. D. (2019). *Socio-cultural differences in treatment of Arab Americans. Professional Psychology: Research and Practice*, 50(2), 93-102.

183.   Bennett, B. E., Bricklin, P. M., Harris, E., Knapp, S., VandeCreek, L., & Younggren, J. N. (2019). *Assessing and managing risk in psychological practice: An individualized approach* (2nd ed.). Professional Resource Press.

184.   Sue, D. W., & Sue, D. (2020). *Counseling the culturally diverse: Theory and practice* (8th ed.). Wiley.

185.   Kitchener, K. S., & Anderson, S. K. (2019). *Foundations of ethical practice, research, and teaching in psychology and counseling* (3rd ed.). Routledge.

186.   Thomas, J. T. (2019). *Ethics consultation in mental health practice. Professional Psychology: Research and Practice*, 50(5), 321-329.

187.   Gottlieb, M. C., & Younggren, J. N. (2019). *Ethical decision making and professional development. Ethics & Behavior*, 29(6), 459-474.

188.   Roberts, L. W. (2020). *A clinical guide to psychiatric ethics*. American Psychiatric Publishing.

189.   Spring, B., & Neville, K. (2019). *Evidence-based practice in clinical psychology. Clinical Psychology: Science and Practice*, 26(1), e12276.

190.   Wampold, B. E., & Flückiger, C. (2019). *The alliance in mental health care: Conceptualization, evidence and clinical management.* World Psychiatry, 18(2), 173-184.

191.   Insel, T., Cuthbert, B., Garvey, M., Heinssen, R., Pine, D. S., Quinn, K., Sanislow, C., & Wang, P. (2019). *Research domain criteria (RDoC): Toward a new classification framework for research on mental disorders. American Journal of Psychiatry*, 176(7), 548-556.

192.   Tapia, G., Laborda, M., Moltó, J., & Baños, R. M. (2020). *Combined schema therapy and EMDR for complex PTSD: A randomized controlled trial. Journal of Anxiety Disorders*, 72, 102-118.

193.   Bisson, J. I., Roberts, N. P., Andrew, M., Cooper, R., & Lewis, C. (2019). *Psychological therapies for chronic post-traumatic stress disorder (PTSD) in adults. Cochrane Database of Systematic Reviews*, 2019(4), CD003388.

194.   Kazdin, A. E. (2019). *Psychotherapy for children and adolescents. Annual Review of Psychology*, 70, 707-733.

195.   Barkham, M., Moller, N. P., & Pybis, J. (2019). *How do we know if our therapy is working? A guide to tracking client progress in therapy.* Sage Publications.

196.   Sackett, D. L., Straus, S. E., Richardson, W. S., Rosenberg, W., & Haynes, R. B. (2019). *Evidence-based medicine: How to practice and teach EBM* (3rd ed.). Churchill Livingstone.

197.   Bernal, G., & Sáez-Santiago, E. (2019). *Culturally centered psychosocial interventions. Journal of Community Psychology*, 47(2), 408-425.

198.   Kazdin, A. E., & Blase, S. L. (2019). *Rebooting psychotherapy research and practice to reduce the burden of mental illness. Perspectives on Psychological Science*, 14(2), 179-194.

199. Lilienfeld, S. O., Ritschel, L. A., Lynn, S. J., Cautin, R. L., & Latzman, R. D. (2019). *Why ineffective psychotherapies appear to work: A taxonomy of causes of spurious therapeutic effectiveness. Perspectives on Psychological Science*, 14(6), 1060-1086.

200. Goldfried, M. R. (2019). *Obtaining consensus in psychotherapy: What holds us back? American Psychologist*, 74(4), 484-496.

201. Norcross, J. C. (2019). *The future of psychotherapy: Introduction to the special issue. Journal of Psychotherapy Integration*, 29(1), 1-5.

202. Reardon, M. L., Cukrowicz, K. C., Reeves, M. D., & Joiner, T. E. (2019). *Duration and regularity of therapy attendance as predictors of treatment outcome in an adult outpatient population. Psychotherapy Research*, 29(5), 673-689.

203. Rosen, D. C., & Davison, G. C. (2019). *Psychology should list empirically supported principles of change (ESPs) and not credentialed therapies or other treatment packages. Behavior Modification*, 43(3), 300-318.

204. Gonçalves, M. M., Ribeiro, A. P., Mendes, I., Matos, M., & Santos, A. (2019). *Tracking novelty in psychotherapy process research: The innovative moments coding system. Psychotherapy Research*, 29(2), 169-183.

205. Baumel, A., Muench, F., Edan, S., & Kane, J. M. (2019). *Objective user engagement with mental health apps: Systematic search and panel-based usage analysis. Journal of Medical Internet Research*, 21(9), e14567.

206. World Health Organization. (2019). *Mental health action plan 2013-2020: Global report*. WHO Press.

207. Hatcher, R. L., & Lassiter, K. D. (2019). *Initial training in professional psychology: The practicum competencies outline. Training and Education in Professional Psychology*, 13(3), 202-210.

208. Koenig, B., & Gates-Williams, J. (2020). *Understanding cultural issues in therapeutic practice: Global perspectives*. Academic Press.

209.   Duran, E., & Duran, B. (2019). *Native American postcolonial psychology*. State University of New York Press.

210.   Lutz, W., Rubel, J., Schiefele, A. K., Zimmermann, D., Böhnke, J. R., & Wittmann, W. W. (2019). *Feedback and therapist effects in the context of treatment outcome and treatment length. Psychotherapy Research*, 29(4), 418-433.

211.   Norcross, J. C., & Rogan, J. D. (2019). *Psychologists conducting psychotherapy in 2012: Current practices and historical trends among Division 29 members. Psychotherapy*, 56(4), 474-484.

212.   Prochaska, J. O., & Norcross, J. C. (2019). *Systems of psychotherapy: A transtheoretical analysis* (9th ed.). Cengage Learning.

213.   Lambert, M. J. (2019). *Prevention of treatment failure: The use of measuring, monitoring, and feedback in clinical practice*. American Psychological Association.

.

www.ingramcontent.com/pod-product-compliance
Lightning Source LLC
Chambersburg PA
CBHW072235270326
41930CB00010B/2145